Our Walls
Life as an Endurance Athlete

Our Walls

Life as an Endurance Athlete

a story about determination in the midst of pain and how you
can choose to move forward no matter how tired you are

Dana-Susan Crews

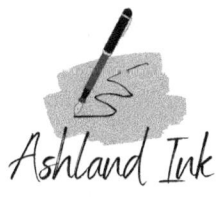

Our Walls

Copyright ©2024 by Dana-Susan Crews
Book design copyright ©2024 by Ashland Ink Publishing

Author: Dana-Susan Crews
Cover Art by Asland Ink Publishing

All rights reserved. No part of this publication may be reproduced, stored in a retrieval system, or transmitted in any form or by any means - for example, electronic, photocopy, recording - without the prior written permission of the publisher. The only exception is a brief quotation in printed reviews.

The opinions expressed by the author are not necessarily those of Ashland Ink Publishing

Published by Ashland Ink Publishing
209 West 2nd Street #177
Fort Worth TX 76102

Published in the United States of America

ISBN: 978-1-963514-00-1 (paperback)
ISBN: 978-1-963514-01-8 (electronic book)

This book is dedicated to my daughter who delights my heart daily and proves that you can rise above the ashes and push yourself with great determination to fight a good fight and finish your race, all while keeping your faith.

CONTENTS

Preface / 10

Chapter 1: A Journey That Changed Me Forever / 12

Chapter 2: A New Lover / 20

Chapter 3: The Dogs Didn't Win / 26

Chapter 4: Ironman Arizona / 38

Chapter 5: Well Done / 54

Chapter 6: Dreams, Slavery, Prison, Glory / 60

Chapter 7: Training / 68

Chapter 8: Rising From the Ashes / 76

Chapter 9: My Wall / 80

Chapter 10: The 12th Mile Marker / 86

Epilogue / 96

"A marathon is a metaphor for life, and life is not easy."

~Meb Keflezighi

PREFACE

I've heard a lot of people say that marathon is a great metaphor for life. True. In fact, many sports are a great metaphor for life, but I think endurance sports in particular are especially aligned with the challenges and obstacles we face in life.

I am an endurance athlete. I have run many marathons and I am an Ironman triathlete. In the more than five decades I've lived on this planet, I have learned how to walk through floods and fires. I have intimately known both the thrill of victory and the agony of defeat.

This book is about the challenges of racing and the pain of living. It is also about the glory of the finish line. I am an advocate for childhood cancer. I am a caregiver. And I am a publisher with a goal of putting a spotlight on cancer in kids and young people. I have learned a lot over the years about endurance. I have discovered that we really can do anything. And I have mostly learned that the journey of life takes us along some super rough roads alone in the dark in great storms, but also through some beautiful mountaintops where the sun sparkles like golden glitter upon the snow.

All things work together ultimately for good if you let them. With the mind of an endurance athlete, I know how to move forward when I'm in agony and I know how to push myself when all I really want to do is lay down and die. Today, I hope you will enjoy some of my thoughts on the race of life and make a decision that you also want to push on 'til you cross the finish line because y'all, that's where the ultimate glory is.

"Our running shoes have magic in them. The power to transform a bad day into a good day; frustration into speed; self-doubt into confidence; chocolate cake into muscles."

~Mina Samuels

Chapter 1
A Journey That Changed Me Forever

𝒜 gentle breeze and the warmth of the sparkling sun greeted me as I stepped out to begin my morning run. I sat on the driveway to put on my Brooks running shoes while my Garmin was trying to catch a satellite. I stuck in my earbuds and found a podcast I thought would be just long enough to last my entire workout, then I pushed the start button on my watch and took off down the street.

It is a scene from my life that could easily represent many of my days during many of my years. Sometimes I run in the rain. Sometimes I run in the cold. Often, I run in the extreme heat of the great state of Texas. Running is simple, yet so profound.

I am a natural born perfectionist. At least I think I am. The argument about nature vs. nurture is too complicated for me, so I don't think too much about it. My parents definitely demanded good behavior, but I think I would have demanded it of myself no matter how they raised me. As the firstborn in the family, I always felt like I had to do everything right and like I had to behave perfectly all the time. I have heard from many other firstborn kids that they are exactly the same way. I took every single thing my parents said to heart. And there were so many things I didn't think I quite measured up on so I constantly felt like a huge disappointment.

At the age of seven, my baby brother got cancer and my tendency to be afraid of germs escalated. To this day, I wash my hands incessantly. I wipe down the counters and scrub the floors even if the maid was just at the house yesterday. I push myself and go to bed almost every night feeling like I could have and should have done more. It is exhausting.

It only made sense that I would end up spending 20 years living in a town that was made up almost entirely of people just like me. Type A perfectionists who pushed themselves in every part of their lives. A beautiful master-planned community north of Houston, The Woodlands is enclosed in trees. Glorious trees everywhere you look. You only know there are grocery stores and restaurants behind them because you live there, but otherwise, every street looks the same. The homes are large. People are wealthy and they drive nice cars. They wear the fanciest of clothes. They work hard and get promoted to the highest of levels. They play just as hard and just as competitively. The town is filled with triathletes and runners and professional athletes of all kinds. The kids in town all make perfect grades. Everyone looks like a model. It is "perfect".

Living amongst perfection only drove me more. I took a daily deep dive into hard work. I did my many workouts and I volunteered for many charities and at my kids' school and I didn't stop working hard from the moment I woke up early in the morning until I went to bed late at night, and it was like that every day. I was happy, but I was exhausted. All the time.

It's not really too surprising that I would ultimately become an Ironman triathlete. It wasn't what I set out to do with my life, but I almost think it was unavoidable. My husband and I had been swimmers and when we first got married, we volunteered coaching a local swim team in the Dallas area. When we moved to The Woodlands, we joined an athletic club where Olympic hopefuls were swimming and diving (in fact, we used to watch Laura Wilkinson who was training there when she ended up winning the gold medal at the 2000 Olympic Games in Sydney).

Almost as soon as we moved to town, people began asking us if we had ever thought of doing a triathlon. After all, most triathletes (at least back then) did not come from a swimming background and they thought swimming was difficult, so they assumed we would be great at the sport since we were such good swimmers. My husband Bill thought the idea of triathlon was brilliant. He always loved a good challenge. He had been very athletic, competing in swimming, soccer, bull riding, baseball, and many other sports his entire life. A new challenge was appealing to him and at first, I thought it would be fun too. Then one of our friends mentioned that the swim takes place in a lake and I was out. The germaphobe in me could not handle the thought of it. Um, no thank you. I am not getting into some dark, dirty lake with duck poop and snakes. No way. Instead, I decided that I would be Bill's biggest fan as he pursued this sport.

It was fun watching him get excited about a new sport. He was really enjoying the running. Cycling was a bit new. We rode our bikes all over town, but not road bikes. We rode on the trails slowly to just be outdoors. Bill is a fast learner, so he was really having fun picking up some new skills . But then he hurt his shoulder. I won't go into that whole story. We did write a book about it if you're interested. But the gist of the story is that his hurt shoulder was cancer. Just three weeks after his 37th birthday, Bill became a patient at MD Anderson Cancer Center in Houston where he was diagnosed with stage four, highly aggressive, completely incurable non-Hodgkin lymphoma that had metastasized to his bones. Instead of doing that triathlon, he got to do chemotherapy.

He was very sick. He almost died. After eight rounds of intensive chemotherapy, he transitioned to maintenance therapy which was much less aggressive. During that time, he did his first triathlon. As promised, I went to watch him and be his biggest fan. But something happened to me that day. I looked around at the athletes jumping into the cold lake and thought, "I gotta do this." So, I signed up for my first triathlon.

That very first triathlon for me was intense. Just as my wave was about to dive into the cold lake in Austin, a woman screamed, "there's a huge snake." She was not kidding. That thing was a monster and it crawled right into the water exactly where we all had to jump in to swim. I was shaking. I was one of the only ladies there not in a wetsuit because I never had worn one and had no idea how cold that water would be. I did not want to get in that water. The snake was bad enough, but then just looking at how rough the water was and how it was pushing the group ahead of ours making it just about impossible for them to swim, I wondered what had possessed me. But when I commit to doing something, I follow through. So, I jumped into the cold water and waited for the start gun.

As soon as the gun sounded, I was attacked by a coughing fit. I was just so cold and shaking way too much and I couldn't stop coughing. I just treaded water for the longest time coughing when one of the lifeguards on the kayak asked if I wanted a rescue. "No," I managed to say and then I forced myself to swim. What an ugly swim. I could hardly see and I couldn't swim straight. But I finally finished that hideous swim and got out of that water to try to run to transition. I could barely walk, let alone run. I was so cold. But I made it to my bike and got on to ride up and down the hills of Austin. Ouch. I shook the entire ride. My teeth were chattering and I realized that I am not a cyclist. Again, I pushed myself and finished. I was so happy to be off that bike and to put on my running shoes.

And boy was that run fun. I absolutely loved every moment of the run. I passed up so many people who had been ahead of me on the bike. I was smiling from ear to ear as I let them choke in my dust. Honestly, it was only a five kilometer run (3.1 miles), but I felt like I could run all day long. I ran at a pretty steady pace of seven minutes per mile (slightly less) and when I crossed the finish line, I found my husband and kids and my mom and sister and said, "I'm gonna do another one." I was hooked.

To make it all even more exciting, we began truly getting involved with Team In Training, the endurance sports campaign at the Leukemia & Lymphoma Society. Bill was still doing cancer treatments, but he kept on racing and every time he crossed a finish line in a triathlon, we felt a huge win over cancer. Then one day, I decided to run a marathon. I had fallen in love with running. I had never known how talented I was at this sport. Early in my life, I was discouraged by running. There were quite a few people in my life who told me that I was really fast, but when I attempted to run around a track, I bonked quickly. I didn't know what I was doing. Perhaps if I had a running coach guiding me, I would have ended up being a runner, but without the knowledge and encouragement to pursue running, I tried a few times and gave it up. I was not about to put myself into something that made me feel like a total failure.

Bill Dwyer changed that for me. He was the Team In Training coach in The Woodlands and he had become a true friend to our family. He had been a long-time marathoner and ultra marathoner and then he became a coach. The first time he ever saw me run was at a track workout. That night, he told Bill that I had the talent to qualify for Boston. He didn't think I would necessarily qualify on my first marathon because I was too inexperienced, but he believed that I had the ability if I continued with the sport.

With his coaching and guidance, I felt pretty confident that I could do this. And because Team In Training is a fundraising campaign, I had another goal besides running 26.2 miles. I had to raise thousands of dollars for blood cancer research. It seemed like a pretty big deal, especially considering the fact that I had two small children at home and a husband who was still doing cancer treatments. Determination kicked in. If I had known how tough training would have been, I might have chosen not to sign up for more triathlons that fall. I was pushing my body way beyond what I could have ever imagined all while being a stay-at-home mom, volunteering for a million charities, and continuing to be my husband's caregiver.

To this day, I still don't think highly of all my accomplishments. You see, while I was doing all of that training, my husband was too. His body had been destroyed by cancer and chemo, yet here he was running and doing even more and longer distance triathlons. Included in that was a half iron distance which he finished in six hours. If the people on the course that day had realized that a cancer patient in treatments was out there racing with them, I can't imagine what they would have thought.

During my training, I injured myself. That's not unusual. Running long distances can be hard on your body and when my iliotibial band began giving me trouble, I didn't rest adequately. Instead, I pushed myself through the pain and ended up getting a bad ankle and knee injury. But I had committed to this race and to the fundraising, so nothing was going to stop me.

January 15, 2006 was a day like none other. My cancer hero and I stood at the start line early that cold day in Houston as the sun began to rise in the sky. It looked like millions of diamonds sparkling above us. I had a bracelet on my arm with the names of 26 people with cancer for whom I was running the race. Each mile was dedicated to someone we knew who had cancer. Bill and I were a combination of excited and nervous. I thought about the fact that we were just a few miles away from MD Anderson Cancer Center and I thanked God for where we were that morning. As the gun sounded and Bill and I began to run, I looked at my bracelet and turned to Bill and said, "this mile's for Chad."

Chad was Bill's college friend who had died at the age of 30 after a two-year battle against leukemia. I imagined Chad and some of the others whose memory I was running for being up there with the twinkling diamonds in the sky. It gave me the boost to begin the journey that would change me forever. One foot in front of the other for 26 miles. I would never be the same again.

"The obsession with running is really an obsession with the potential for more and more life."

~George Sheehan

Chapter 2
A New Lover

On January 15, 2006, I crossed the finish line in my very first marathon in Houston, Texas. In those days, I did not wear a watch like most runners do. And that day was my first marathon so I didn't want to be worried about my time. All I wanted was to finish the race. Those last two miles had been especially challenging. I was in so much pain from an iliotibial band problem that had caused an ankle and knee injury that I was almost limping. In fact, at the mile 24 marker, I hit a wall. My wall wasn't a glycogen depletion. My wall was cancer. My wall was the sudden welling of emotion of running this race for 26 people I knew with cancer, including my own brother and my husband who was out there somewhere on the course (at least, I hoped he was still out there). I had been fighting cancer for so long. And this race was not just a marathon. It was a battle against cancer.

My wall was enormous and I hit it hard. I was wearing my Team In Training singlet and my name was written on my race bib. Additionally, I was wearing a purple hat that read "For Bill". It was obvious to any of the people out cheering that day that I was running for a guy named Bill and that he very likely had cancer. Five young women were standing on the street cheering for runners when one of them saw me hit my wall. Her eye caught my eye and I stopped. I stood there for what felt like an eternity, but was really only a few seconds. Then she quietly started chanting, "Go Dana."

"Go, Dana. You got this."

"Come on Dana, do it for Bill, Dana."

She got louder and louder and then her friends joined her. They were all chanting loud. "You can do this, Dana. Do this for Bill, Dana. Run, Dana. Go. For Bill. For Bill. Go, Dana."

It was all I needed. With their chants, they blew that wall down and I ran. I hurt like Hell, but I ran. I put one foot in front of another and I told cancer to flee. Moments later, a Team In Training coach from Oregon found me and began to run alongside me. He was very kind and kept trying to encourage me. I kept asking if he knew where Bill was. I was so concerned about him out there. He told me he wasn't sure where Bill was, but that he had no reason to be worried and neither should I. He told me to just keep moving because I only had two miles to go. I told him that I had a lot of pain in my knee and ankle and at that point, my feet were burning too. I had never run that many miles. The most we had done in training was 21 so this was all virgin territory for me. I didn't realize my feet could feel like they were on fire and I didn't see how I could finish.

I didn't say much to this coach, but every so often I would say, "I just want to finish." He kept saying that I would. Then before long, I saw the final mile marker: 26. It was beautiful. I looked up and noticed the finish line ahead. I heard the music and the noise and longed to be there. I had no idea that the final point two of the marathon was so excruciating. The coach told me that he was going to let me cross the finish line on my own. He said that I deserved that glorious moment. This was something I would never forget and I practiced that same thing when I eventually became a marathon coach. Let that athlete cross that finish line alone and soak in the glory of their finish.

Since I wasn't wearing a watch, I had no idea how long it had taken me to run this race. When I crossed the finish line that day, I looked up at the big clock and the very first thing I thought was "Oh, wow, I just qualified for Boston." Immediately after, my second thought was, "Crap, now I have to run another marathon."

Glory. That was exactly what it felt like. The medal around my neck. The long walk back through the convention center to get to the Team In Training tent. The exhaustion. The pain. The Boston qualifying time. The thousands of dollars raised for cancer research. Glory.

I had heard from others that crossing your first marathon finish line is emotional. I am pretty good with words, so when I tell you that I have no words to describe it, that's because it isn't possible. I think I would have been emotional even if my husband didn't have cancer and I hadn't been raising all that money and running each of my miles for cancer patients we knew. But when you add all that together, you get a pile of emotion that cannot be explained. I suddenly began to cry. I sat in the tent with a banana I couldn't eat and tears poured down my face. I had just turned 36 years old. I have never before or since been proud of myself. But that day, I was proud of my accomplishment. I even bought the race photo and it's hanging up in my home as my most favorite photo of me ever taken. I sometimes look at that photo and think, "I am so proud of you, young lady."

Seven minutes after I crossed the finish line, Bill did. Again, what would the other folks out there running that day think if they knew that someone doing cancer treatments had just finished a marathon in less than four hours? He came over to the tent and hugged me. We were overjoyed. We were so thrilled. We had no family out there cheering us on that day, but we realized that the Team In Training community was our family and they always will be.

Three months later, we flew to Boston and I ran my second marathon. I obeyed Coach Bill Dwyer's command to "just enjoy". He told me to go slow and run each mile at about a nine minute pace. So, I wore a watch to make sure I obeyed. By doing this, I was truly able to soak it all in and enjoy Boston. I loved every minute of it. From Hopkinton to Boston, I high-fived kids and waved at the folks cheering along the way. I smiled the entire race and talked to other runners as we made our way through the streets where marathon is life and part of the great tradition of this amazing city. Turning down Boylston Street and crossing that finish line was a thrill. In my old life, I had no idea I could qualify for this race, let alone go out and actually run it. It was the icing on the cake of a season in my life that had been much-needed. I had a new lover. Marathon.

"I don't run away from a challenge because I am afraid. Instead, I run towards it because the only way to escape fear is to trample it beneath your foot."

~Nadia Comaneci

Chapter 3
The Dogs Didn't Win

It wasn't a big leap to go from running marathons to competing in a half iron distance triathlon. But I knew within about 30 miles on that bike that I don't like cycling at all. Normally a half iron triathlon includes a 56-mile bike ride, but this one was long by three miles, so I ended up riding 59 miles through some beautiful national forest. However, several of those miles were along stretches of road with potholes and torn up streets. I did not enjoy it at all and by the time I started the half marathon, I was in a bit of a bad mood. I was also not feeling great and couldn't take in nutrition. When I crossed the finish line, my blood pressure was very low and I almost fainted. This would be the first of a few trips in my racing life that I got to hang out in the medical tent after crossing the finish line.

Bill and I were scheduled to speak at an event for the Leukemia & Lymphoma Society that evening and we had to rush to leave the race site and get cleaned up to head over. Neither of us had eaten all day long and we had just completed a big race. I'll never forget the looks on the faces of the staff at the event when they saw how weak we looked. Thankfully, they were able to get us something to snack on before we spoke and then we left early to go to dinner. I was a tiny woman, so I could tell the wait staff at the restaurant was shocked to see how much I could eat.

Training and racing multiple marathons and triathlons over the next several months and years was not just a recreational activity for Bill and me. These races were our way of fighting cancer. And not just for him, but for everyone with cancer. We became so close to the other "honored teammates" (people of every age who were battling blood cancers and letting the Team In Training participants race in their honor).

Our children were becoming pretty great little athletes too. They were on a local swim team and when Dylan was only four years old and Morgan had just turned seven, they did their first triathlon. They would go on to finish several triathlons that were specifically designed for kids and our family motto became "You don't have to win, but you do have to tri." These were fun, happy days for us. In fact, we had so much fun that often we would forget that Bill was still undergoing treatments for cancer.

Well, we forgot that is, until we walked through the doors of MD Anderson Cancer Center for another ten-hour infusion. Actually, if I'm honest, there were daily reminders. The therapy Bill was doing was depleting his B cells where his cancer originated. Our B cells are a critical part of our immune system. They have a "memory" and let the body know which antibody to create to fight specific infections. The constant killing of his B cells meant that Bill had to endure constant colds and flu-like symptoms. If the people racing against him knew how sick his body was, I think they would have been shocked. After all, he looked like a professional athlete out there racing.

In addition to his current therapy, one of the chemo agents he had done during intensive chemo, doxorubicin, causes a lot of damage to the heart. And Bill reached his lifetime limit of doxorubicin. He had a lot of cancer, so he had to take in a lot of chemo to kill it. So, when he began talking about doing an Ironman triathlon, I asked him to wait. I was his number one support for all the other racing, but when it came to a race like the Ironman, I needed him to finish all of his therapy first and get one year past it. He agreed. He would finish therapy and one year later, he would do an Ironman.

Bill finished his almost three years of cancer treatments in the summer of 2006. There would be some additional treatments for him later, but the main therapies were complete and our job now was to go back to a protocol that is called "watch and wait" because his cancer is incurable.

What were we watching and waiting for? For his cancer to attack again.

The following summer, around August of 2007, Bill called me from work. It had been a year since he finished cancer treatments. We had raced in many marathons and triathlons, but he kept his promise to me about the Ironman and waited. When I answered the phone, he said, "I am on the website for Ironman Arizona and they only have a few slots left."

To this day, I cannot believe the words that came out of my mouth, "Ok, sign me up too." As soon as I said that, I wanted to take it back, but he immediately hung up the phone. Ten minutes later, I got an email that said, "Congratulations. You are registered for the 2008 Ford Ironman Arizona." Crap.

Now you have to understand that what I said earlier was still true. No matter how much I enjoyed the overall sport of triathlon, I still did not like the cycling. And I had figured out why by this point. I love swimming. I have a background in swimming and it is the only sport that makes me feel clean and fresh and strong and it has a healing effect on my body and soul. I had fallen in love with running too. Before I became a marathoner, I didn't understand how people could run for so long and not get bored. But I learned that the long run was just as healing to my soul as swimming. It was fun running with friends, but even alone it was uplifting. Those moments out on the road moving my body gave me peace like nothing else ever had.

But the bike. That was my nemesis. With swimming and running, I was using my own body to move. There was no equipment necessary, just me and my body. A bike is technical. Not only do you have to have special shoes and aero bars (that's a triathlon thing), but you have to have special tires and you have to know how to change gears and how to get into an aerodynamic position and in this sport, to have a high cadence and conserve your hamstrings for the run. You have to know how to change a flat tire quickly by yourself because of the "no outside assistance" rule. It's work. It's dependence on a piece of equipment instead of just your body.

There are so many athletes who love the bike. Triathletes, in particular, seem to truly have a love affair with their bikes. They talk about them more than any other aspect of the race. They get aero bars and aero helmets and Zipp tires and they spend thousands and thousands of dollars on these things. It exhausts me. Instead of bringing me healing and peace like swimming and running, it brings me a headache, almost like doing Algebra problems. Yuck.

But I was registered for an Ironman now, so I had no choice. I bought a beautiful Quintana Roo bike. She was blue, my favorite color. She was super pretty and helped me go super fast. Our race would be in April and we had about nine months to prepare. Because Bill and I were both racing and because we had two young children at home with no nanny, we had to take turns training. We both knew that we would not be performing our best since we couldn't train the way we needed to train, but we were doing this to become Ironmen, not qualify for Kona. Training was going fine. It was a cold, damp winter and a lot of our cycling had to be done indoors on a bike trainer and that was horrible. Running had to be done outdoors in terrible weather. So, I wished that I could just swim all the time. But honestly, the swim was getting annoying too because I was mostly doing long distance swimming at the pool and only doing freestyle. I was perfecting my bilateral breathing as it was supposedly going to help me swim in a straight line even if I couldn't see the buoys.

In fact, the late, great coach Dick Bower gave me a few lessons in breathing that I will always remember. He was the swim coach to trust. He had coached athletes in four different Olympic Games, including in the 10-kilometer open water "marathon" swim. "Don't forget that you need lots of oxygen for a long distance swim," he told me. He said he preferred breathing every stroke, but he understood my desire for bilateral breathing and told me to breathe every three strokes. That rhythm helped me so much on the race.

In March of 2008, I agreed to join an all female team to run the very first Texas Independence Relay. This consisted of two days and nights of running over 200 miles through Texas. We were a team of 12 women and we had two men who drove two vans full of us and all our gear. We each had designated legs of the relay to run. On this inaugural event, there were some strict rules. One of those was a "no shadowing" rule, meaning that the vans couldn't follow you along as you ran. They had to go ahead and meet each runner at the next spot where we would tag the runner who would go next.

On one of my running slots, it was a perfect day. It was about 3:00 in the afternoon. The sky was deep blue and the air was dry and crisp, not hot and not cold, but just right. All I had to run were three little miles from one tiny town to the next. Unlike a marathon or a typical footrace where you are surrounded by other runners, this one was all spread out because each team started at a different time. So, there I was all alone on a long highway in the middle of nowhere. Because I was only running three miles to the next little town, I didn't keep my phone with me. Three miles is easy and I would be done in about 20 minutes so the van of teammates left me and waited in the next town.

About a mile into my run, I heard dogs barking. It didn't phase me at all. I had a beautiful dog at home. I have always had dogs and I love them. Barking dogs as I ran through farmland on a lonely Texas highway just seemed natural. But soon I realized that I might be in danger as the barking got louder. I looked to my left and a gate was cracked open and three dogs were barking and growling and running through the gate directly toward me. Immediately, I regretted not having a phone. I also wondered why no one had thought of bringing pepper spray. I was literally alone with no weapon and no phone.

One of the dogs was little, probably less than 20 pounds. He was the loudest of the three. The other two outweighed me. All of what I am about to describe happened quickly, but I will write it in slow motion. I prayed that God would help me. I knew I was in trouble. I couldn't imagine how this could possibly be the way that my life ended. Running along a highway being slaughtered by dogs was not the way I wanted to go. The little dog kept up the noise while the two big dogs surrounded me. One was in front of me and it put its paw on my throat. I knew it was about to slit my throat and kill me. The other one went behind me and bit me on my butt. Then it bit me again. Somehow, I was able to keep myself standing and then I heard the voices of two men yelling at the dogs to get off of me. They obeyed. Two huge men came running toward me from the home inside the fence. One of them grabbed the dogs (they were his dogs) and went to lock them up inside a shed. The other man told me that he was there visiting his friend when they heard the commotion from the dogs. He saw the blood gushing down my leg and said, "why don't you come into the house to clean up." Uh, sure. I'm gonna walk inside of some house in the middle of nowhere with two men I don't know.

"No," I said and then I pointed at my race bib and said that I was not allowed to move from my spot because I was in a race and it was against the rules. I asked if I could borrow a mobile phone to call my teammates. I told him they were right down the road and that they would be really worried about me and that they were probably on their way to get me and would be there at any moment. I wasn't about to have my life saved from the crazy beast dogs only to then have these men assault me. Maybe they were nice guys, but I wasn't about to find out.

The man handed me his phone. I realized that I have no phone numbers memorized other than my husband's and he was hundreds of miles away in The Woodlands coaching swimming. But I had to call him and ask him to call my teammates. I was so glad he answered his phone. He doesn't usually even hear it when he's on deck coaching. As soon as he answered, I said, "I need you to stay super calm and do exactly what I'm asking." I told him a dog bit me and that I needed him to call our friend Bill Dwyer and ask him to call Debbie on my team and let her know I had been bitten and was hurt. Somehow, Bill managed to stay calm and do exactly what I asked. I hung up the phone and the owner of the dogs came out. I showed him where I had been bitten twice and he saw the bites and the blood. Then I said, "The black dog bit me. Does it have its shots?"

"No," said the man followed by, "I think he just scratched you". Dude! I have teeth marks on my butt and blood flowing down my leg. Your dog better not have rabies!

You know that God is real, right? I do. I was standing on the highway with two men I don't know and dog bites from a dog that hadn't been vaccinated. I am on a 200-mile race event that is super spread out so when I tell you that God was with me, I mean He was right there on that road. Out of nowhere, an ambulance showed up on the highway. It was the ambulance secured by the race officials to monitor the race and out of 200 miles, it just happened to show up exactly where I was on a long, country road. It was flying by at 60 miles per hour and then stopped and turned around to come toward me. I will never forget one of the men saying "Looks like your husband called an ambulance for you." Seriously? I talked to my husband two minutes ago and somehow he managed to call an ambulance and without knowing where in Texas I was, he was able to get them here in two minutes? Dude!

The EMTs got out of the ambulance and walked over to me. Almost immediately, the two men disappeared. They got in a car and drove away. One of the EMTs said, "we were heading toward the next town and saw you standing there in a race bib and that scene didn't look right." Wow, thank you Jesus for sending me help!

I told them what happened and they got me into the ambulance to clean me up. It wasn't hard to do. The bites were deep, not wide, so although it hurt really bad, there was no need for any stitching as it was not a big slice. They gave me some antibiotics and while they were cleaning me up, my team showed up as did Bill Dwyer's. Everyone was panicked until they saw that I was fine. The sheriff arrived and questioned me before they broke into the shed to haul the dogs off to quarantine them. He said they would be quarantined for two weeks and if they did not have rabies, they would let me know. At that moment, all I could think of was the fact that I was six weeks away from racing Ironman Arizona and I might have rabies. I was mad.

One of my teammates picked up where I left off on the run while another of my teammates and her husband stayed with me. The EMT said there was a hospital up the road and he wanted me to go get checked out just to be safe. My teammate and her husband took me to the hospital as we were instructed. I checked in at the ER and told the nurse exactly what had happened. I told her they gave me antibiotics and that the bites were deep, not wide and that even though it hurt, I thought I was fine.

Although the door to the exam room was now closed, I heard the doctor outside my room say "Why is she here? What does she want, a Bandaid?" What a total jerk. He then came in and said, "There is nothing we can do for you" and left. The nurse made sure to let me know that she was certain that the dogs who attacked me would be killed because I had called the sheriff. I did not call the sheriff. I did not even call the ambulance. I did not show up at the hospital because I thought they could do anything. I was following orders. I paid $200 to be treated like a total fool and they were sure to condemn me for "permitting dogs to be killed". Just to clarify, the dogs were not killed. They were quarantined for two weeks and then sent home and side note… the following year, they almost attacked another runner, but thankfully, the race directors had changed the "no shadowing" rule because of what happened to me and that runner's team was there to protect her.

I left the hospital angry. How dare that disgusting "doctor" treat me like a hypochondriac! I was limping and already noticed that my entire hip and butt were turning black, but that anger pushed me. I called my husband who was in the car with our kids driving toward me and told him to turn around and go home. I was not going to be dropping from this race. Those dogs were not going to stop me and neither was this pitiful excuse of a health care team. Fear and pain would not hinder me from finishing the Texas Independence Relay and it would not keep me from Ironman.

My next leg of the race was supposed to be that night, but there was no way my teammates would permit me to run until they knew I was better. And we no longer cared about the rules. The vans would stay near the runners from that point on. It wasn't right for women to be out there alone during the day or the night. Worse things than dogs could have been out there. It was funny that I sort of became "famous" out there. At our next several aid stations, I heard people talking about the "girl who got attacked by dogs". A photo of my butt ended up on the internet too, but that is another story all together.

Later in the race, even though my whole hip and butt were swollen and black, I ran (slowly) and didn't let the dogs destroy my running career. To this day, I take a stun gun with me when I run. Too many people walk around with their dogs unleashed. You know your own dog and you might think that your dog is friendly and wouldn't hurt anyone, but I don't know your dog so if you don't leash your dog and I'm out running and I get scared, you better know I have a stun gun and I will use it.

My hip was in quite a bit of pain for several days, but I had a race to train for so I didn't take any time off. I was grateful two weeks later to get a call from a sheriff letting me know the dog that bit me did not have rabies. I kept pushing my body and trying to maintain my weight. My normal weight is 105 pounds, but with all the workouts I was doing, I kept slipping under 100 pounds and for some reason, this scared Bill. He was afraid that if I got too thin, I would not have the strength to finish Ironman. So I ate and ate and ate in between my workouts. In those last few weeks before Ironman, I must have been eating 5,000 calories every day and I couldn't just go out and eat donuts. I had to eat foods that would enhance my performance. I learned that bananas and avocados have a lot of calories so I ate them a lot. And I was doing really great about staying at 105 pounds.

Then just three weeks before Ironman, I got strep throat. I had never had it before. My throat felt like it was on fire. I almost never get sick. Why was this happening when I had such a big race in just three weeks? My doctor gave me a shot of penicillin and a bottle of penicillin to take. Because Bill had virtually no immune system, he was also put on penicillin. He felt fine and was able to mostly continue to workout, but I was in bed barely able to move. And I could not eat. If Bill had not been so worried about my weight, I would have not cared, but because he was so concerned, I had to drink chocolate milkshakes from Whataburger. Yeah, not healthy, but it was all I could handle.

Bill and I finally made our way to Arizona. At check-in, the first thing we did was get in line to be weighed. Back then, they weighed all of the participants and put their weight on the back of their bib. Bill was right behind me in line. I was so nervous. I was wearing the heaviest pants I owned and the heaviest shoes I could find and hoping they wouldn't make me remove them to weigh. They did not. I stepped on the scale and the woman called out, "she's 105". Whew.

I have written about my Ironman race before. My race report is out there on the internet and I will write it again in its entirety in the next chapter. But, this is the important takeaway from this chapter: don't let anything stop you. When you are preparing for something big, there will be many obstacles. The best things in life don't come to us easily. And the glory of the finish line is way more glorious when you had to go through much torment to get there. The dogs didn't win.

"Dana-Susan Crews from The Woodlands, Texas, you are an Ironman."

~Mike Reilly

Chapter 4
Ironman Arizona

The following is from my personal journal, written in April 2008

Thursday, April 10

We arrived in Tempe, Arizona. Sunshine, blue skies and dry air greeted us. As we drove down Rio Salado Drive and straight toward Tempe Beach Park, immediately we saw the Ironman tents. It was quite thrilling just to be in the atmosphere of this big event. We walked passed the finish line and entered the athlete village where we stood in a small line to pick up our packets. First they handed us a paper and we had to check off a couple of things and sign it. Next we stood in line to be weighed.

Our next stop was at a long table where we were handed our bags filled with all the essentials. There were the transition bags and special needs bags. There was the timing chip and multiple stickers with our bib numbers to place on the bike, helmet, running belt and the many bags. There were detailed instructions and a schedule.

After scanning our chip, Bill and I walked around for a while through the Ironman Village. First thing I wanted to see was Town Lake. Someone who had done the swim that morning informed us that the waters were so dark you couldn't even see your own hand right in front of you. We were also told the temperature was 65 degrees. Yikes!

Once we bought a few M-dot items, we left and checked into our hotel. We spent the evening mostly relaxing. We ate at Monti's and got to bed early. As I quickly drifted off to sleep, I thought about how cool it was that we were finally here. It was like a dream and I could hardly believe that it was really happening.

Friday, April 11

Today started with a quick breakfast and then we were off to the Gatorade Practice Swim at Town Lake. There were a few hundred people doing the practice swim. Any time from 8-10 a.m. Ironman athletes were allowed to jump in and give it a try. We started at 8 sharp. I just wanted to get it done. I stuck my toe in first. Cold. But I quickly warmed up with the sun beating down and wearing my nice Team In Training wetsuit. I was happy to see a few others with Team In Training suits on too. I realized that on race day I would be starting my swim about 200-300 yards back so I'd end up swimming way more than 2.4 miles. Some people did not enjoy swimming directly into the sun for that first mile, but I discovered that the sun kept me warm and gave me something to sight on. I could not see the buoys, but I could see the sun rising over the bridge. I only swam about 400-500 yards out before turning around. On the way back, I realized I could easily get lost. I could not sight well. But the truth is, just taking a small swim on this beautiful Friday morning was really amazing. It is all part of an incredible event. Ironman is not just one day. It's many months of training and then several days of excitement. I'm in those days right now and I don't want to forget a moment of it.

After the swim we showered and ran out to buy a battery for my Cat Eye computer on my bike. We also had lunch and then headed back to the Ironman village for shopping and to meet up with Jon and Jill who had arrived from Colorado. They did some shopping too and then we all headed to Iron Prayer.

Iron Prayer is held at most Ironman events and it's a great time to hear some inspirational stories from Christian triathletes and have a prayer time. All of the speakers were wonderful. They included last year's Ironman champion Heather Gollnick who reminded us that we do this for God's glory, the president of Fellowship of Christian Athletes Endurance and a super Ironman athlete and coach from Phoenix. But I think I was most inspired by the young man who didn't let losing his arm stop him. He's an Ironman who swims with one arm, but I'm sure he'd beat me with my two arms. Although he's done many Ironman events, his next adventure is the Ultra Man. I can't even wrap my brain around that one.

After Iron Prayer, we headed to the banquet and mandatory athlete meeting. We saw some of our Woodlands triathlete friends there. We did some carbo loading and watched some cool videos and listened to some speakers including of course, Mike Reilly, "the voice of Ironman". Bill and I were excited to also hear Frank Farrar get up and speak some. He's someone we've been wanting to meet face-to-face for more than a year. He phoned in January of 2007 and told me he'd read an article I'd written in a magazine. He told me he was a lymphoma survivor who'd done 25 Ironmans. By the time I hung up with him, all I knew was that he was a banker and lawyer from South Dakota who owned four planes and usually flew himself to Ironman events. Later I "Googled" him to discover he was also the former governor of South Dakota. Since then, Bill has kept in contact with him through phone and email. Finally tonight we got to meet him and his sweet wife. Frank will do Ironman with us on Sunday. He's 79 years old and filled with energy and he's one of the most delightful people you'll ever meet.

Saturday, April 12

This day was tough. I was so sleepy all day and terribly emotional. It started with a phone call from the kids. They were doing well, but Dylan started crying because he missed us so much. Then Morgan started. It made getting through the day hard for me, being Ironmom first and Ironman second.

We ate breakfast before heading to transition with our bikes and bags. The only bags we turned in this morning were swim-to-bike and bike-to-run. Then we turned in our bikes. Once everyone had done that by 3:00 p.m., it was amazing seeing millions of dollars worth of bikes in transition.

Bill and I ate some really good pasta early afternoon and a small supper later. We went to bed early with great anticipation about tomorrow.

Race Report
2008 Ford Ironman Arizona
Tempe, Arizona
Sunday, April 13, 2008

THE ARRIVAL:

The alarm sounded at 4:00 a.m. and we had some coffee. Slowly we dressed in our tri kits before heading down for a yogurt and bagel. Ironman hopefuls filled the breakfast area in the hotel, nervous and excited for the long day ahead. Bill and I went back to our room and grabbed our special needs bags, morning dry clothes bag and wetsuits. We prayed for the day and got in the car, driving through the dark morning, arriving at the parking garage by 5:00 a.m. What a busy place it was as thousands of athletes and their very dedicated families and friends walked down to the Ironman village.

First stop for us was special needs bags located about 300 yards from transition. We dropped off the run special needs bag and the bike special needs bag. Then we made our way through the huge crowd to the transition bags to drop a few more items in them. Next, we went to our bikes. That's where we separated for a while. Bill's bike was on the opposite end of mine. My bike was in row 27 where I quickly met several women and enjoyed a few moments of talking and laughing. I helped one lady pump her tires. She had borrowed Zipp tires and was struggling with the pump. Together we wore ourselves out, but got the air in. That was my warm up for the day! Next I pumped my tires, then got body-marked.

Bill and I found each other again and found a place to sit near the bikes and just relax for a few minutes. That's where we saw our friend Greg Goedeke. He had slept well and was ready for the day. We thought it was great that he had done more than just train; he had taken it a step further and used this as an opportunity to raise funds for the Leukemia & Lymphoma Society.

It was interesting to just sit and watch everyone. Some of these people were "Iron Virgins" as they called us Friday night. They were pretty nervous. Others had obviously done many Ironmans before. There was a young man to our left doing yoga poses and "relaxation" techniques. There were many who were talking loudly and laughing. Others were grouped together doing light stretching. Many of these athletes wore happy faces. But there were some who seemed to take the day more seriously than others (and I'm not talking about the professionals). Some of these guys with their big M-dot tattoos had the intense look of a charging bull. I thought, "They better not be near me in that swim." But the coolest part of all was that right there in one transition area were age-groupers and pros. What other sport on the planet has that? Here we were, amateurs, right there on the same playing field as the professionals. In the same transition area. With the same rules. Facing the same mileage.

THE SWIM (2.4 miles)
At 6:30 the professionals crossed the line and started jumping into the lake. They were allowed to start 15 minutes before us to try to keep the swarm of swimmers off for at least a few minutes until some of the really fast age groupers caught up. While the pros treaded water, the rest of us crossed the line. Bill and I crossed with our friend Mark Tefft from Lone Star Multi Sport. He looked relaxed and ready. I kissed Bill one last time before stepping down on the pier. I knew I would not be kissing him for many more hours. I was completely calm, not an ounce nervous and so glad about that. For three weeks before this race I was nervous and sometimes even a little frightened. Three weeks before this day I was in bed with strep, taking penicillin and even the day before I was exhausted, feeling like I might not even make the swim, let alone the entire race. But now, there I was on that pier at the 2008 Ford Ironman Arizona

surrounded by more than 2,000 athletes and thousands of fans. No anxiety. Just peace and a lot of joy to be there. I eased my way to the cement side of the lake. The water was cold on my feet, but I wanted to wait as long as possible before getting completely immersed in that water. I didn't want to spend 30 minutes treading water. I talked to all the athletes around me. Finally no one acted superior. We were all in this together. We were all facing a 2.4-mile swim through very dark, cold waters heading for the first 1.5 miles directly into the sun. At 6:50 a.m. I finally decided to get all the way in the water. Knowing where to position myself was impossible in that moment. All I could see were thousands of swimmers. Some wore blue caps (the men) and others wore pink (us girls). I treaded water and looked ahead only to realize I could not see anything but the big, bright sun. That would be how I would sight because looking for buoys or bridges would be impossible. At 6:55, the national anthem was sung and the crowds got louder. Mike Reilly, the "voice of Ironman" got them pumped. "Today, you will be Ironmen," he screamed out over the mic. We blue and pink caps looked like bobbing heads til he said that. Then suddenly our arms were up in the air and our voices screaming in zeal for the big day.

Boom! The cannon sounded and the swim began. Within minutes a man had kicked me so hard in my face that my goggles slipped off, filled with water and my vision was even worse than before. I had to stop as many swimmers kicked and stroked right over my body while I fixed the goggles. I thought, "Y'all won't get away with that nonsense," and I passed them all up. But it would not be long before I realized, of course, I had no idea where I was. I was in a pack of crazed swimmers, many of whom were kicking way too hard for wearing wetsuits. I just told myself to swim slow and steady and not let their anxiety influence my swim. I knew I was facing a 112-mile bike in the heat and wind. I knew I would need my upper body strength to endure that, so why waste it on over-swimming? I never got away from the pack through the whole swim. So I was kicked often and hard. Going into the sun was tough, but I wasn't as bothered by it as others were. Once we turned around, it was easier to sight off the orange buoys. I was able to swim a little faster, but never got too fast for fear of tiring out. When I saw the last buoy, I was thrilled. I very slowly and carefully let the volunteer help me up the steps. Then the next volunteer grabbed me and began stripping me. I was shaking terribly and she asked if I needed medical. "No, M'am," I said with chattering teeth, "I'm just cold." She handed me my wetsuit and I lightly jogged to transition. I grabbed my bag and ran to the changing tent.

SWIM-TO-BIKE TRANSITION

Here's where I must describe the volunteers. They are amazing. There were 3,500 of them out that day. They treated us like rock stars. I've never felt so pampered. It took me a while in the changing tent just to dry my feet, put on my socks, bike shoes, helmet, gloves, sunglasses and drink some water and Gatorade. I didn't have to do anything with my wetsuit or clothing. The volunteers took care of everything. I ran out of the changing tent and a volunteer was standing there with sunscreen. He rubbed it all over my face, arms and legs. I didn't have to do a thing! I went to the port-a-potty and then ran toward my bike. I grabbed my bike and ran to the mount line, hopped on and began the longest, toughest bike journey of my life.

THE BIKE (112 miles)

The meteorologists had predicted 6-10 mph winds for this day. They were wrong! And those people who think the Ironman in Arizona is flat are wrong! The bike course is three loops including a long 15-mile stretch of straight, slight uphill through the Pima-Maricopa Indian community. I was no longer cold from the swim. It was approaching 95 degrees. The winds unfortunately were not tail winds up that hill. There were moments when I could feel the wind pushing me backward down the hill and I had to tap into my core muscles to control the bike. It wasn't long before I saw people falling. I saw people crashing at the turns as the winds and sharp turns wiped them out. The heat was unbearable. I talked to the Lord and asked for strength to endure. If loop one was this challenging, how on earth would I endure loop two and even more difficult, loop three?

I saw Bill heading down the hill as I was getting toward the top. We screamed out to each other. That was a little boost for me. I think he was happy to see me too and know I was still in the race. I was pretty good at throwing away my water bottles and grabbing fresh ones from volunteers at the aid stations. I was not taking food from them. I had brought along pretzels and fig bars in my Bento box. But I really couldn't eat. I was extremely nauseated. It wasn't long into the bike that I started seeing people on the side of the road vomiting. It would happen over and over again for the rest of the day. I saw more crashes and more vomiters. I soon found it just about intolerable to refuel. I had trouble stomaching the Gatorade and craved water so desperately. But out of fear of possible hyponatremia, I took the Gatorade and sipped it through my aero bottle. Of course I was covered in salt and Gatorade and sand for most of the trip. Then around mile 40, I was covered in grease as my chain fell off the bike and I spent five minutes trying to get it back on. My fingers weren't functioning well. A teenage volunteer was so nice to me. I had no wipes or tissue, so he literally gave me the shirt off his back to wipe off my fingers. "The only way you can repay me," he smiled, "is to win this race!" I guess I owe that young man a shirt!

It was probably about mile 50 when I realized a DNF (did not finish) was highly possible. In the wind and heat I could not get my cadence up. My whole body hurt (partly from taking penicillin and partly from months of training) . My shoulders ached from the swim and the constant having to hold on tight to keep from falling in the wind. It didn't help me any psychologically to see so many strong athletes on the road wounded. Later I would find out that this particular Ironman event had the third largest DNF rate in the history of Ironman with 17% of the athletes not finishing. Most of those who did not finish were taken off the bike course, never even making it to the marathon. Now I realize how blessed

I am that I was able to endure. The bike is my weak part. But when it comes to wind, I'm a big baby! I kept asking myself, "Why do people say this is fun?" There were a couple of times when I actually got all the way down to seven mph going up hill into the wind. Exhausted and ready for a nice shower and nap, I made it to mile 56 and thought "Wow, only 56 more to go and then a marathon!" Welcome to Hell, DS!

My favorite part of the bike course was the area near the finish which was hard to approach when I knew I wasn't on the last loop. The fans there were loud and encouraging. They said things that I knew were horrible lies, but I loved them for it. Things like, "You look strong, Girl" or "Way to go Iron Woman!" All along, I kept looking at my watch reminding myself that if I didn't make it to loop three by 3:00 p.m. I would be disqualified and removed from the course. As I was finishing up loop two, I knew I'd make that cutoff, but loop three of that course was probably the hardest thing I've ever done in my life. With sand and dirt and grease and sticky Gatorade all over me and lips so chapped they felt like they were on fire, I pushed and pulled and exhausted every ounce of strength left in me. I spent the majority of my time praying, but I must admit I spent a little of that time cursing the wind! I told my bike, "I love you, but I don't want to see you for the next six months!"

Finally I got to my last big turn around and headed downhill. This time I didn't push myself at all. I just coasted. My legs, my tooshie, my whole body hurt. A volunteer let me use her chapstick after I came out of the port-a-potty at the final aid station. A couple of the aid stations had run out of water by now and I was forced to sip Gatorade which was making me nauseated. I craved water. I could tell I was dehydrated. As I hopped back onto my bike, happy to be nearly finished with the ride, I wondered how on earth I would manage running a marathon. With about eight miles to go, a panicked biker passed me by and asked, "When is the bike cutoff?" I told him it was 5:30 and he seemed suddenly very relieved as he said, "Oh, thanks, I thought it was 4:30."

Soon I was back into town. I passed by Sun Devil Stadium and the crowds had thinned out. But then I got to the finish sign, turned right into the chute and the crowds were cheering me by name (it was on my bib) which was nice because none of our family or friends had been able to come cheer us on at the race. A volunteer grabbed my bike. I removed my shoes and realized my feet were burned and blistered on bottom. They were also pretty swollen. I walked across the timing pad and grabbed my bike-to-run bag.

BIKE-TO-RUN TRANSITION

Just before I got into the changing tent, a volunteer said, "Your husband said to tell you he's about 15 minutes ahead of you." I thanked the nice man for letting me know and I thought about how proud I was of Bill being out here doing this event. I was relieved to know he was still in the race. There were obviously many others who had not made it.

I hobbled into the changing tent and a volunteer quickly took my bag from me, began emptying it and helped me sit down. She asked if I needed medical attention and I smiled and said no. I told her I needed a few minutes to rest. She brought me a cup filled with ice and a few pretzels. The ice was exactly what I needed. I don't think I have ever been that hot. I saw my friend Nora Wilson in the changing tent. She had crashed on the bike (thanks to the intense wind). Her leg and arm looked awful. She was badly bruised and swollen and had finished her bike ride using only one leg. Being the incredibly strong lady she is, she would go on to run the 26.2 miles to complete another Ironman.

I changed from my tri kit into running shorts and shirt. The volunteer asked if she could put my shoes and socks on for me. I told her I could do it. I did. Then I put on my Team In Training hat and sunglasses, left my gear behind, and walked out where another volunteer rubbed me down with sunscreen again. I felt very dehydrated as I made my way to the run course.

THE RUN (26.2 miles)

There were spectators everywhere here and they were truly delightful. As usual, my favorite fans were the kids. They always hold their tiny hands out for a high-five and no matter how bad I feel, I always smile as I high-five them and thank them for their encouraging cheers. "You look good Iron Lady," screamed one little girl. I missed my kids so desperately in that moment. The first aid station was right outside of transition so I stopped. I took a sip of water and a few sips of chicken broth, but nearly puked. I couldn't imagine doing a marathon. My feet were covered in blisters. From the top of my head to the bottom of my feet I was in agony. But I did not endure the torture of nine months of training to get out here and DNF after a 2.4-mile swim and 112-mile bike. I was going to finish this thing no matter what!

The run course was three loops. The sun was still blaring and I was walking. Unlike the swim and bike, though, on the run I was able to talk to people. That was my "savior". I met people from everywhere. Some were on their second or third loop, but others were afraid of not making the time cutoff because just like me, they had just begun the marathon. I encouraged them, telling them that they could definitely walk the whole thing and still finish. We had started at 5:00 p.m. Our cutoff for the run was midnight, although we had to be at loop three by 10:15 or we'd be disqualified and removed from the course. At the next aid station, I grabbed the cold wet sponges and drenched myself. Next I took a cup of crushed ice and another sip of chicken broth. I held on to the crushed ice and for the next several minutes, I kept it in my dry mouth. I loved meeting people and actually found myself trying to encourage those who were struggling to finish. Often I felt like "Coach DS" out at the Houston Marathon and in many ways that kind of distracted me from my own pain. I stopped at every aid station on the run course. I tried sipping the cola to see if it would help with the nausea. It did not. I tried eating oranges and cookies. That made me sicker. All I wanted was water and ice and took it more and more. I know it's important to keep salt in your system in that kind of heat, but I was so sick. Soon, I couldn't even tolerate the water and at the aid stations where ice was available I just took ice.

As I was finishing up loop one I saw Greg. He was slowly working on loop two. Soon I saw Bill again. He slowed down hoping I'd catch up, but I told him he shouldn't do that because I was pretty far behind. Again, I was so glad to know he was still moving. The thought occurred to me that my wonderful husband was soon to become an Ironman. How proud I was!

When I finished loop one and came back in where the finish line was, it was painful and not just physically. I couldn't bear hearing people cross the finish line when I knew I had two more loops to go. At the aid station I stopped and sat on the ground to empty my shoes of the rocks. One of the spectators sat next to me and asked if this was the beginning of the run loop. I told her it was. She asked if I was on my last loop. "I wish," I smiled as I put my shoes back on. She kindly smiled back and wished me luck. "You are doing great," she said.

I kept running into a lady I'd met who was from southern California and doing her first Ironman. She was terribly nervous about making the cutoff and I kept trying to assure her that her pace was fast enough to do it. Every time I saw her I smiled and told her she was still on target. I think I was trying to make myself believe that too, but I was getting a little concerned that I might not make it either. Finally it was dark out and I was glad that the sun was no longer beaming into our faces. I put my sunglasses on my hat. I continued walking as fast as I could. On the downhills, I lightly jogged a couple of times. But I can now tell people I know what it feels like to basically walk a marathon. My run was slower than my walk. I actually passed many people who were running and realized that the walk muscles were just working better on this night. As I began loop three and realized I had nine miles to go, I met Jen from

North Carolina and we stayed together for about three miles. She and I had made the third loop by 9:00 so we were safe. We would have three hours to finish and we knew that we could do that. I thought about the fact that finishing was now quite probable and longed to cross that finish line. But I now was hurting worse than I ever have in my life. Even my eyes were burning. I wondered how Bill was doing and wondered if he'd finished. I continued encouraging the people around me. I continued seeing people on the ground vomiting. I could no longer tolerate even the water so the only reason for going to aid stations now was to see if they had ice and go pee if I could.

There were many little hills and they were torture. The fans on the streets were mostly gone by now and the darkness brought on some loneliness. I've heard the quote many times and finally it made perfect sense: "There's no 'I' in team but there is in 'Ironman'." Now I get it. It was just me out there. There were many others struggling to get through it around me. But I was the only one in those long, dark moments who could push myself to go on. Even if I had family or friends out there cheering for me, they couldn't have forced me to finish. That was up to me and me alone. I did not want to fall, but I was getting dizzy and the nausea I'd felt for the past 15 hours was getting stronger. I kept telling myself that vomiting was ok, but the last thing I wanted was to faint or drop out now. I had two miles to go and limped through that aid station. One of the volunteers asked if I needed medical. "No," I softly answered. I was determined not to need medical on this race. I wanted to finish and not to have to be taken to the medical tent even at the finish line.

At mile 25 I felt relieved. Only one mile to go! I passed by a man who was limping. "Are you ok, Honey," I asked. He painfully answered no and I said, "I know how you feel, but keep going. You will be an Ironman in one more mile."

With great pain and nausea, I walked furiously toward the finish line. I could hear the music and the fans, the incredible noise and longed for it. I turned left and there were the volunteers screaming "Go Girl, you're 200 yards from becoming an Ironman". I turned left again and there was the finish line! There was Bill screaming my name. There was that chute I'd longed to see for nine months. I decided to run across the finish line. Then I heard the words I'd waited for. I'd endured 16 hours of torment just to hear those glorious words and when I did, I felt nothing but relief and joy and a depth of satisfaction like words cannot describe. "Dana-Susan Crews from The Woodlands, Texas, You are an Ironman!" I shot my arm up in victory. A volunteer put a medal around my neck. Another volunteer handed me a finisher's shirt and cap and asked if I needed medical. "No," I victoriously smiled, "I'm fine, thank God, I'm fine!" There was Bill grinning. I grabbed him and kissed his cheek. "You're an Ironman, Bill," I smiled, "I'm so proud of you!"

"I'm so proud of you too," he smiled. We had our photo taken together. We grabbed some pizza! We sat and wondered if we'd be able to get up again.

THE DEPARTURE
I couldn't tolerate food. I ate a piece of pizza, but hated it. It took a while, but soon we got our bike and transition bags and walked back to the parking garage. It seemed like it had been a week ago that we were parking in that garage. We returned to the hotel. I checked my emails and discovered that several of our friends back home had actually stayed up to watch the live feed online and saw us become Ironmen. Houston time that would have been 1:00 in the morning when I finished and 12:30 when Bill finished. What incredible fans we had at home!

I showered and that was my most favorite time of the day! I crawled (almost literally) into bed. As I drifted to sleep, I thought about Bill. I think Ironman probably has a depth of meaning for him that most people out there racing don't get. He survived cancer and now he's an Ironman. I love him!

Next morning, we attended the breakfast and award ceremony. We sat with Mark, Raul, Nora and Dana Lyons. Dana is a USAT coach and incredible athlete. He had done his first Ironman this weekend too and qualified for Kona. His wife was there too and she was so proud of him. We stayed to watch him receive his award. Then we grabbed our DVD and certificate and walked back to transition one last time to pick up our special needs bags. My bike one was missing so I just got my run bag.

Then we left the Ironman village. As we left, I realized what we'd accomplished. I don't know if I'll ever do it again. Finding time to train is nearly impossible. The race itself is grueling. I know recovery will take some time. But I don't have to ever do it again. I'm an Ironman! It is finished. And like they say, "The pain is temporary, the pride is forever!" To God be the Glory!

"Well done, good and faithful servant."

~Matthew 25:23

Chapter 5
Well Done

So, I never in my life intended to run a marathon or complete an Ironman. Life took me on a most unexpected journey. My journey consisted of extreme sickness and extreme health. I regret none of it. But something had changed permanently in me because of the extremes. My brain changed.

Having always had the attitude of "go big or go home," it made perfect sense that I would become an endurance athlete, but what I did not expect was that it would change the way I view exercise forever. To this day, if I "only" swim 2,000 yards or "only" run five miles, I feel like a failure and like I haven't done a thing. I feel like I have not earned the right to eat if I have "only" spent an hour lifting weights. Endurance sports changed the way I think and I don't believe there is any way to go back.

I have attempted to retrain my brain. I have forced myself to read articles about normal physical activity, especially for women my age. But the endurance athlete in me has a stronger voice than any of those articles.

And this "malfunction" in my brain extends to everything else in life, not just health and fitness. No matter what I do, I put everything into it and refuse to rest until I'm done. Actually, I have a tendency to not rest then either because I always begin the next big thing right away. Sure, I have always been this way naturally, but becoming an endurance athlete was a way of feeding the monster. I feel like a lazy bum if I'm not super busy working hard all of the time. And this has worn me out. So before I continue, I want to say something very important. Rest is essential. And by the way, it is also an action word. You aren't doing nothing when you rest. You are doing something. And the something you are doing is absolutely one of the most important things you can do. So, do it.

In fact, as a woman of faith, I love the fact that God Himself taught us the valuable and essential necessity of rest by doing it Himself. He spent six days creating the universe and then on the seventh day, He rested. I don't think He rested because He was tired. He rested as an example to us that we need to rest too. The action of rest is one I preach to athletes when I train them. The issue is reminding myself to practice what I preach.

Extreme. That's my life. It is extreme. I don't know how to have normal daily troubles. Major, life-altering troubles somehow find me. Extremes in both the positive and negative find their way into my life. And lately, I have found myself wishing for calm. I want to know how to just sit on a pier at the lake sipping on a latte and just relaxing. I want to know how to go hiking at my favorite park without worrying about my speed or heart rate. I want to jump on a pair of roller skates and just skate around the lake by my house like a kid. I want to be satisfied if all I do for "exercise" in the day is take my dog on a walk. I want to think it's ok to eat even if I didn't workout. I want to dance in my kitchen while I cook and find just as much joy in that workout as I do in a 10-mile run. But I can't. Not yet. I am a work in progress, y'all.

I literally am in a situation in life in which I don't have to do anything if I don't want to. I don't have a job. I have been an empty nester since 2018. But instead, I find myself working hard volunteering for multiple nonprofit organizations and pushing myself harder than ever. People with that kind of mentality get a lot done. I'm not mad that I am the way I am. We are the type of people who take visions and dreams and make them happen. But we are also the type of people who are never satisfied as we are always longing for that next big thing.

Many years ago, I was in a crowded airport as a hurricane was approaching. All flights were being canceled and we were waiting for someone to pick us up to take us to a hotel, hoping we would have electricity and make it through the storm. The airport was a huge mess with passengers on the floor waiting for updates on what to do or for transportation to a hotel. I sat on the floor with my husband and kids looking around at everyone as they ate and talked and complained. It was super noisy and filled with commotion. Then I turned and happened to notice how full all the garbage bins were. Trash was everywhere. People couldn't get their garbage into the bins as they were full, so next to each bin were piles of disgusting trash. Then I saw a woman who was part of the custodial staff walk over to one of the bins with a large plastic trash bag. She looked about 70 years old. She was short and a bit frail with a tiny limp as she walked. People were all around her as she made her way through the crowds on the floor to get to the bin to empty it. No one noticed her. She was invisible to them all, even when she said, "excuse me" to try to get through them all. They couldn't hear her or see her.

I watched her for a bit and noticed something really remarkable about her. She was smiling. Here she was at her age, in this crowded airport filled with trash, unnoticed by any human around her, yet she was smiling. Why? Did she like her life and her job that much? At the time, I had just published my first book and I was anxious, wondering if I would make it to my scheduled book signing event. I was tired from traveling and wishing for a nice shower and my bed to sleep in. I understood all the whining and complaining coming from folks all around me. Yet, here was this unnoticeable woman emptying trash bins with a smile. No one talked to her or saw her, yet she didn't seem to be bothered. It hit me in that moment that there was Someone who saw her. Did she know that? Did she know that God was watching her? Was she smiling because she knew that God was proud of her hard work? Was that knowledge enough for her to go on and do this job at her age? Even if no one else notices your work, is it enough for you if God does?

That moment helped to shape me. I work so hard all the time and most people have no idea what all I am doing. But God knows. He sees me. And if I am working for Him, does anything else matter? This thought also has made me realize that all of the "go big or go home" ideas of mine mean nothing unless God is with me, seeing me. He is not quite as impressed with what I do as I might be. Yes, that Ironman was hard to do and I did it and I'm pleased, but God created my body that did it. That's way more impressive. Whether I am emptying garbage bins in an airport or crossing finish lines in races, I have decided that I want my head to hit the pillow every night with the most important words spoken from God: "Well done, good and faithful servant."

I cannot change the way my brain works thanks to endurance sports and life, but that 70-year-old unnoticed woman in the airport lobby emptying garbage bins is my hero and inspiration. I want to do everything that I do for God's glory. And I want to do it with a smile. That is the only way for my life to mean a thing. I hope that woman went to bed that night (assuming the hurricane didn't wipe out her home) hearing the words "well done, good and faithful servant."

"You can't be brave if you've only had wonderful things happen to you."

-Mary Tyler Moore

Chapter 6
Dreams, Slavery, Prison, Glory

I might not be the best at teaching valuable life lessons. I am not writing this to do that. This is just a bit of a glimpse into the life of an endurance athlete and how those sports represent my life. If you can learn anything from my ramblings, great. Otherwise, I hope these words will at least entertain you a bit. Or maybe you'll be turned on to the idea of running a 5K or trying a new sport. I promise that you will not regret it. But through this little book, I also hope you will learn the value in hard work followed by some rest.

No matter what, I believe that each of us has a purpose for being here. Yes, there are billions of people on the planet. No one is more significant than anyone else. It is easy to disagree with me on this. You might think that the president of the United States matters more than that woman in the airport, but I don't. Without that woman, we'd all be sitting in piles of garbage.

Do you remember the story about President John F. Kennedy and the janitor? No one seems to be able to validate the story, but I love it anyway. President Kennedy was visiting NASA and learning more about the work to land on the moon. While there, he walked into the restroom and a janitor was in there. The president asked the janitor what his job was at NASA and the man replied, "I'm helping to put a man on the moon." You see, from the highest level at the company to the lowest, all the positions matter. Some jobs are easier than others. But all the jobs matter and must be done.

Because I believe that we all have a job to do, I work hard on what I believe is my job without comparing it to anyone else's job. One of my most important jobs in life was to raise my children. It was also the hardest job I have ever done. It was the most rewarding too. Additionally, it's been my job to raise funds for cancer research and to do advocacy on behalf of cancer patients and their families.

Just over 20 years ago, I knew I would have another job. I was given a "vision" and even though I wanted to leap into that job, I wasn't ready. I needed to be trained and that training was some of the toughest training I have ever done. In fact, I can tell you this without a doubt… all the training you do for a marathon or an Ironman is way harder than the actual race. Way harder.

But before we dive into the training, I want to share about a man in a story who has inspired me greatly. His name was Joseph and he was the next to the youngest son of a man named Jacob (whose name was changed to Israel). If you have ever read the Old Testament of the Holy Bible, you probably know this story well. If not, here you go…

Joseph was his dad's favorite. Now, I'm a parent and I don't understand having favorites, but I have heard from many other parents who say they do have favorites. Perhaps it's because I have a daughter and a son, I don't have a favorite. My daughter is my favorite daughter and my son is my favorite son. At any rate, it seems like having favorites is probably not healthy for the kids, but Jacob had a favorite and it was Joseph. He pampered him and bought him a coat that was filled with colors which at the time was a big deal because dyes were expensive.

Joseph was a dreamer. And before I go deeper into this tale, I will say that there were many other dreamers mentioned in the Bible which is why I don't think we should put down dreamers. By this, I mean the people who have dreams and visions and then later, they see those come to fruition. I don't mean people who just sit around dreaming, but never do anything about it. Joseph had a dream that signified that his brothers would bow to him. I think he probably should have kept that to himself, but he told them about it anyway. They were obviously super annoyed with him and that annoyance had built up over time as they watched their dad love him a bit more than he loved the rest of them. So, finally, they came up with a plan to get rid of their brother. They decided to sell him into slavery and tell their dad he had died. They stripped off his colorful coat and dipped it in blood to make their dad believe he had been killed by an animal, but really he had been sold as a slave and carried away to Egypt.

While in Egypt, Joseph gained the favor of the pharaoh and got promoted quickly. You see, in addition to being a dreamer, he was also diligent and worked hard even as a slave. This has always stood out to me as a great example of how we can all be. No matter our circumstances, we can work hard and that might lead to a promotion. Sadly, this didn't last long for Joseph though because the pharaoh's wife wanted Joseph to take her to bed. He refused her and then she pretended that he had been trying to get her into bed which obviously ticked off the pharaoh who threw him into prison.

Joseph was in prison for a long time. He was unjustly sold into slavery and then unjustly thrown into prison. He didn't deserve the stuff happening to him. I wonder if he ever thought about that dream he had years before. I wonder if he ever questioned God. Meanwhile, at one point while he was in prison, he met the former baker and butler of Pharaoh. Both of them had dreamt something and they told their dreams to Joseph. Now, Joseph wasn't just a dreamer of dreams. He was also an interpreter of dreams. He told them that God was the One Who gave him the interpretation. In the case of the butler, Joseph told him the good news that his dream meant he would be set free from prison and go back to work while the baker's dream meant that he would be hanged. I imagine the baker was not too happy to hear that. Meanwhile, the butler promised Joesph that he would remember him once he was freed.

Well, in just a few days, the butler was set free and the baker was hanged on a tree. Sadly, the butler forgot all about his promise to Joseph. So, there sat Joseph in prison. He had done nothing to deserve the horrible things that had happened in his life. I know too many people who are super judgmental and see people in circumstances like Joseph's and think "that guy must have done something bad for God to let that happen." Wrong. Very wrong. I don't claim to know how Joseph was feeling during all of this, but I'm sure he wondered why this was happening to him.

Then two years later, Pharaoh had a dream and it bothered him greatly. He desperately needed an interpretation of his dream and no one could give it to him. That's when the butler remembered Joseph and told Pharaoh about him. Joseph was taken out of prison to give him the interpretation of his dream which basically was that the land was going to have seven years of plenty followed by seven years of a great famine. Pharaoh was so happy to know this that he set Joseph free from prison and put him in charge of saving up food during the seven years of plenty so there would be more than enough during the famine.

In fact, Joseph became second in command in the land of Egypt. And because of his hard work, food was saved during that first seven years so that when the famine struck, Egypt had way more than they needed. Then folks from other places journeyed to buy food from Joseph. Included in that were his brothers. All but one of his brothers was sent to Egypt by their dad to ask for food. The one brother left behind was the youngest, Benjamin. He and Joseph had the same mom, Rachel. When the brothers arrived, it had been so long since they had seen Joseph that they did not recognize him. He did recognize them though. They bowed before him just as he had dreamed. Instead of revealing himself to them, he pretended to not understand their language and through an interpreter he asked them if they had any other brothers. They told him that they had a brother at home and one who had died. Joseph said that he would not give them food unless they brought their youngest brother with them.

So, they left and returned with Benjamin and not long after this, he finally told them who he was. There were many tears shed. The brothers had so much regret for what they had done and pleaded with Joseph for his forgiveness. He replied something I will never forget. He said that they had meant it for evil, but God used it for good. Often in life, I feel like things have happened to me that were meant for evil, but God used them for good.

Joseph had to wait a long time for his dreams to come true. And during that time, a lot of horrible things happened to him and a lot of great things happened too. His dream finally came true, but Joseph had to endure much waiting before he would see it. Like Joseph, I have had dreams. In 2002, I had a dream and vision of children with cancer writing children's books and I was there to help them. At this point in my life, I had experienced cancer many times. As a child, I saw my brother fight cancer. Over the years, I knew friends who fought cancer and just the year before, one of my former coworkers had died of bone cancer. Through the years, I had always wanted to do more to help people battling cancer, especially children. When this idea popped into my head, I fell in love with it. I had a dream and a new mission, a job to do and I just had to do it. But like Joseph, I would end up having to go through some excruciating life circumstances and a lot of years to get to my dream.

One year later, my husband was diagnosed with cancer. I was worn out from the journey. There were times that it felt like our family had been thrown into prison unjustly. And there were many times when it felt like the butler had forgotten us there even though he promised to mention us when he had been set free.

My journey to starting a publishing company was long and dark and difficult. There were many victories along the way though too. I don't complain about the hardships and challenges even though they have left me with some scars. I find myself being thankful for both the good and the bad times and I truly believe that all of those things can and do work together for good. Every step of the way in this journey of life, I have discovered that endurance sports are the best metaphor for my life and probably for yours too. From the burning feet at mile 24 to the being alone in the dark at Ironman to the other racers and fans cheering us on to the music and noise at the finish line, life is one big race. And just like I learned through my racing adventures, the more pain and anguish you feel along the way, the greater the joy and glory of the finish line.

"All progress takes place outside the comfort zone."

~Michael John Bobak

Chapter 7
Training

Endurance races are challenging and quite difficult. But the training is even harder. In March 2003, Bill and I took our kids to Spain to visit my parents. They lived in Tarifa, the southernmost town in Europe. Their condo was on the beach and when you walked out onto the balcony, there was Africa. We had been there before, but this was the first time we had taken our kids so we went on several fun European and African adventures with our parents and kids.

One evening we sat in the parlor at my parents' home and I told them about my idea for a publishing company that would publish books by children with cancer. We also told them that we had a big heart for young people with cancer like our friend Chad who had died that January at the age of 30 after fighting leukemia for two years. We didn't know how it all would happen, but we really wanted to do this and felt like it was our calling in life. My parents encouraged us and told us they thought this was a great idea. On the way home, as our plane got closer to Houston, I remember looking out the window and having this strong feeling that soon Bill and I would be heading to MD Anderson Cancer Center.

Boy, was that right. In October, Bill got cancer and we were caught in a great whirlwind. My mom told me she would help take care of my kids while I took care of Bill. My dad was able to come to the States too, but also had to travel back to Europe for meetings. Our whole family had to fight. I needed them and I needed my friends. I remember early on in this war my dad saying that he thought this was our "training." Bill's cancer was like going to school to become educated on that calling of ours to start a publishing company and help young people with cancer.

I hoped that this training thing was for both of us and not just for me. I prayed often that if God was training us that He wasn't training me to understand and help widows because I did not want to lose my husband and I definitely wanted my kids to have their dad.

Gosh, my dad was right. We learned so much. We could have never truly understood what families go through unless ours had endured this. Cancer was bad. Chemotherapy was worse. We were so exhausted from the constant warfare that I wondered if we would even make it to a finish line. Like I said, training for a race is harder than the race itself. It takes months of great determination and discipline. There are days you have to get up at 4:00 in the morning and rush off to meet someone for a run in the sleet. There are days when you have worked hard and you're exhausted, but you still have to go to the natatorium and swim 4,000 yards. Eating is even a struggle because you have to treat food like fuel and feed yourself the right things and the right amounts.

The training in life is hard like that too. There are nights when you put your ear on your husband's chest all night long to make sure he's breathing. There are 2:00 in the morning vomit fests and you can't just stay in bed for hours later because you have a 7:00 appointment in the medical center. There are infections that land your best friend and the father of your children in the hospital barely alive and you're pleading with God to save him. If you want to know more about our cancer training in those days, you can read that book, *A Time to Fight*. Meanwhile, while we were training, I didn't always think about our dream and vision. In fact, I don't think I ever did. I was too busy being a caregiver.

So, when Bill did his first triathlon after intensive chemo and we got involved in Team In Training, it started to become clear that our dream was coming true and that it was not going to look at all like we had thought it would. How does marathoning and triathlon racing equate to publishing books? Well, again, I tell you that all things work together for good.

I had written a special book for Bill with the kids. I took the words of Morgan and Dylan and created a little book for their dad called *Our Daddy's Cancer, How We Helped Him Fight*. We presented it to him for Father's Day and he loved it. He showed it to so many people at work and to his friends and soon, people were asking if they could have a copy for someone they knew who had cancer and who also had small children. Through our now deep involvement at the Leukemia & Lymphoma Society, the patient service manager also asked for copies of the book to distribute. Eventually, I sent the manuscript to a publisher and it was published in 2007. This was not how I imagined we would get our foot in the door and start publishing books and materials, but that's how God chose to make it happen.

Not long after that, we published our original book called *A Time to Fight* just for the Leukemia & Lymphoma Society to distribute at patient education conferences. Then I began writing various articles in magazines and health journals. We got very actively involved in advocacy, speaking with legislators about blood cancer research and we were also volunteering with programs at MD Anderson Cancer Center.

Then in 2008, shortly after Ironman Arizona, Bill became part of a national ad campaign for MD Anderson. They put him in magazine ads and on billboards and commercials on television. Our kids were in the ads too and so was I. Later, they also did a documentary about him. His determination to get up after cancer and take back his health was inspiring people all over the country and even the world. We got actual fan mail. One was even from the governor of our state, Rick Perry, who was a triathlete too. I didn't keep all of the letters, but I did keep the ones from kids. They were adorable. An article written about Bill in *Runner's World Magazine* was used by a teacher in North Carolina and a lot of her students wrote Bill fan mail telling him that he inspired them to stop complaining about life and get up and do something big. It truly was remarkable.

Toward the end of 2008, I wanted to put together a party to celebrate because on January 26, 2009, we would be celebrating five years of remission. Bill's disease was not cured, but we could still celebrate the fact that he was in remission. Instead of just a party, I decided to host a fun run and I presented my ideas to my friends Jon Walk and Bill Dwyer. They know everybody in the running community and I knew they could help. The night I met with them, I had mentioned this to another friend and when she showed up, it was was just so sweet because it lifted my spirits. Her name is Lisa Henthorn and I just had this strong feeling that she would be with me through to the end.

In fact, it didn't take long before a host of people I love, including my family and friends, joined forces with me and the Bill Crews Remission Run was created. We raised thousands of dollars for a tissue bank at MD Anderson. We hosted the event for five years and a lot of amazing stories that could fill the pages of many books were shared with us. We met some truly incredible cancer warriors and our lives were changed.

Hosting the event each year was not easy. It was a full time job for which none of us was paid. And although I will always remember the good, I can definitely say that there were moments I just didn't see how we could make it happen. We were hit with some of the craziest weather. The event was so detailed and over-the-top because well, like I said earlier "go big or go home." In the end, those were amongst the happiest days of my life and I will be eternally grateful for the gift of being a part of something so impactful.

It wasn't long after we did our final Remission Run that I found myself working full time at the Leukemia & Lymphoma Society. None of what I was doing seemed to be leading toward starting a publishing company, but I knew I was working with cancer patients and fulfilling my calling. I was motivated to go to work full time at the LLS when one of our honored teammates, Andy, relapsed with leukemia. Andy had originally been diagnosed at the age of two and after four years of treatments, he was doing well. But when he turned 10, he relapsed and it was a nightmare come true. I was angry. Angry at leukemia. It is an evil monster that attacks children and I hate it with the strongest and deepest of hatred.

On my very first day of full time employment there, I learned quickly that one of my reasons for being there was my friend Sue Van Natta. Sue had been raising funds through Team In Training for decades and she had raised $100,000 and run multiple marathons. Her nickname was Super Sue because she was super. I will never forget the hilarious things she said on our long runs or the way she encouraged everyone around her. In her late 40s, she was running faster than young people in their 20s. Every marathon she ran was a Boston qualifier. She was so strong and fit and healthy and always so very loving to the cancer patients at Team In Training. You know how sometimes in life it feels like you've been punched in the gut and you can't breathe? That's how I felt when I got the call that Sue had cancer. And she didn't just have early stage, easy-to-treat cancer. She had invasive breast cancer and five months later, she was dead.

When I took my job at the LLS, I knew immediately that I wasn't just there for Andy. I was also there to honor Sue. I created a team with Sue's daughters Rachel and Rebekah called Team Super Sue and the goal was to get lots of Sue's old running buddies together for a Team In Training event at the Houston Marathon. I had many emotions during that season. Andy's battle was a tough one that lasted for a long time and Sue's memory was honored, but at the same time, I felt a hole in my heart. Things were both good and bad. Do you see how life goes? Good and bad.

Training. All of this was life being lived and callings being fulfilled, but it was also training. You see, the publishing company was still in my heart through it all. I was just way too busy raising my kids and working and volunteering and I was too tired to make it all happen. I needed to keep waiting and hoping that the right time would come. Like Joseph, my wait would be a long one. Until it happened, I kept on training.

"I have tested you in the furnace of affliction."

~Isaiah 48:10

Chapter 8
Rising From the Ashes

I dreamed about lions. They were outside my home ready to pounce. Most of them were in the front yard. In the back, crouched behind the pool, there were wolves. So, I couldn't go out front or lions would eat me and I couldn't go out back because there were wolves. This wasn't just one dream. I dreamed it many times. Then I lived it.

Not all of our family stories are ones I'm free to share publicly. I can tell you that for us, there are worse things than cancer. I can tell you that the extremes I mentioned earlier happened. The protective wall around us was broken. If I thought that my husband's war on lymphoma was bad, I had no idea what bad was.

One of the "lions" got my daughter. A "wolf" got my husband. My son and I had to watch in horror, unable to do a thing about it. Because of ongoing legal battles, I cannot tell these stories. I will simply say that justice was not swift and I'm not sure we will ever get real justice at all.

What happened to my daughter when she was a teenager was cruel and it shattered her. She was harmed and I had no idea how to fix it. This was on the heels of my husband becoming a whistleblower in a serious matter. Our family was unsafe and if affected us all in different ways. We could have easily been completely demolished, but I am proud to report that we rose from our ashes. We saw what appeared to be the total destruction of our family more than once, yet we rose.

Today, I wonder why we had to suffer so much. There is a place in my soul called the furnace of affliction and we have been in that place. Usually I think that adversity produces strength. But I learned that affliction can produce great and enduring pain.

So, what do you do when you are filled with pain and that pain cannot be eased at all? Do you lay down and die or do you rise? Do you rise and walk fiercely even though you are in pain? Yes. Do that. Rise. Walk fiercely. Stand. When you get knocked down, stand again. And again. And keep on doing this, my friend.

When the lion and the wolf attacked and I wasn't allowed to talk to anyone about it, I remembered my Ironman when I was alone out there in the dark. No fans were out cheering even though I knew my loved ones were praying for me at home. No one was there to hold my hand. I had to go on by myself. When the lion and the wolf nearly killed us, I was screaming in agony alone. I reminded myself to get up. Are you bleeding and filled with pain? Get up. A finish line awaits. You cannot see it now and you cannot hear that lovely music or all the cheering from fans who love you and crossed before you, but it's there, my friend. It's there so get up. Move. Walk if you cannot run. Crawl if you cannot walk. But move forward! Get to the glorious finish line and you will see that it was worth every ounce of pain you were forced to endure. When that crown is placed on your head and that booming voice says "well done," you will know that all the struggles of the training and all the hours of the long and difficult race were worth it. The finish line awaits you so please stay in the race. You can do this.

Ashes. That is what is left after the fire is out. You are choking in the ashes and you can barely breathe. The furnace of affliction is hot and not everyone survives it. But if you are one of those who has survived, if you are sitting in the ashes, please don't give up. You might not be able to rise quickly. You have been shaken to your core. You are profoundly hurt and you feel forsaken. So, if you must, sit there for a bit. I know you're choking on the ash, but don't move too quickly because you might fall. So, sit. While you sit, pray. Pray for strength to rise. And then, rise. If you fall into that ash again, that's ok. Sit for a bit. Pray. Then rise again. Do this over and over and over again if you have to. The point is to rise.

Eventually, you will find the strength to walk out of the ashes. And guess what! There may be a day when you are finally able to open your eyes and you will see beauty right there where those ashes were. In place of the furnace of affliction, you will see flowers and trees and children playing and friends celebrating. You will laugh again and you will dance and you will soak up the glorious rays of the sunshine as they shine upon a perfect day. Trust me, I know. You might have many more years in the furnace. You might have a long wait in the ashes. You might have miles and miles to go before you cross your finish line, but choose to rise. Choose to move forward. Choose to finish strong without a DNF. The day is coming when we will all celebrate a glorious finish line together. Every tear will be wiped away and every pain will be lifted. I promise. It is coming. I have seen it in my soul and it is beautiful.

"Obstacles don't have to stop you. If you run into a wall, don't turn around and give up. Figure out how to climb it, go through it, or work around it."

~Michael Jordan

Chapter 9
My Wall

In 2020, I was working at Make-A-Wish Foundation and like everyone else, I thought the lockdowns would last for two weeks and that we would be set free again. So, even though it was heartbreaking to have to tell kids they couldn't have their wish yet, we all thought it was very temporary and very fast. Of course, that was not the case.

Around the summer of 2020, I was becoming very disheartened by this. I had spent decades raising awareness and funding for cancer research and I had taken the position at Make-A-Wish in hopes that I would get to be a part of something fun and uplifting, a more "feel good" side of the childhood cancer problem. But because of COVID, well, that turned sour. So, I began strategizing on a way for me to leave my job and get back to my first passion which was bringing an end to cancer. Finally, in December I resigned. And almost immediately I told Bill that I knew our time had come for publishing children's books written by children with cancer.

We had moved to Fort Worth in 2018 when our youngest went to college, so we were empty nesters. The publishing industry had changed dramatically since we first had our vision. Our first step would be to create a limited liability company and for that, we needed a name. When I thought of the beauty for ashes mentioned previously, I knew right away that I wanted to incorporate the word "bella" in our name. It means beauty and I think of cancer as the furnace of affliction these kids endure and I want them to find beauty for those ashes. But Bella what?

The star is a meaningful symbol for me. When I was a baby, my parents called me the Number One Star Baby of the Universe which often was shortened to Star Baby. I am from the Lone Star state. I love the Dallas

Stars hockey team. And in fact, I love more than any other thing, to lay on a blanket out in the country looking up at stars in the midnight sky. So, I wanted the word star to be in our name. I wanted the kids who wrote books for us to shine like stars in the sky. But Bella Star just didn't feel right. Then it hit me.

My grandma died of cancer when I was 14 years old. Her dad left his home in Greece to come to America, but that Greek blood runs deep. So to honor my grandma in Heaven, I chose to use the Greek word for star which is "asteri". And well, it went great with Bella, right? So, Bell Asteri Publishing & Enterprises was born.

Our first books to publish would actually be a republishing of two of our original ones. In January of 2020, we had been given the rights to our books and with that, permission to republish second editions if we wanted to do so. So, we republished *Our Daddy's Cancer, How We Helped Him Fight* with updated artwork done by Morgan and bylines in both of our kids' names as we had originally wanted it to be. Then we condensed our book *A Time to Fight* and published a second edition.

Quickly, we began talking to our many contacts in the childhood cancer community and started signing contracts with authors. Some of those authors were parents of kids with cancer, some were siblings of kids with cancer and others were the kids with cancer themselves. Some were children's books while others were novels. Things were moving quickly.

I was reconnected with a woman I adore. Laura Eicher is the director of childhood cancer initiatives at the American Cancer Society. She heads up a program called Gold Together and she asked if Bill and I would like to serve on the National Advisory Council for Gold Together. It felt like we were coming full circle. Both of us had been siblings of a child with cancer. My brother survived his disease, but Bill's sister died of her leukemia at the age of six. We knew this was the right fit. Finally, all the years of training and all the years of hard work had led us to the original dream. Twenty years. That's a long time to wait for a dream. All the years of hard work during those 20 years, well that was not how we would have planned it. We would have preferred to jump right over Bill's lymphoma and all the hardships and head straight into publishing the books and serving on this great council. But if we had jumped over all that, we would be worthless. We needed every bit of that pain to make us the people we became.

There were a lot of days when I wanted to quit. During those decades of training, I had mental and emotional breakdowns. I had physical pain. It was one struggle after another. I am glad we didn't drop out of the race. Bell Asteri is hard work. We don't get paid for it. Instead, we invest a lot of Bill's hard earned money to make it happen. So, why are we doing this? We do this because it's our calling. In fact, I would say it's our wall.

There is another old story that comes to mind. A man named Nehemiah was living in exile, but he was Jewish and he had it in his heart to rebuild the wall in Jerusalem. He was granted permission from the king to go and build the wall, but he faced much adversity and opposition as he tried to make it happen. No matter what he faced, though, this was his passion and he wasn't going to give up. He fought long and hard to do what he believed was his calling, to build the wall.

Cancer was my wall. It was my wall to overcome and my wall to build. Way back at mile 24 of the Houston marathon, it was my wall to overcome. It was my wall when I was a seven-year-old child with a brother with cancer. It was my wall in the most heated and difficult moments at Ironman. It was my wall for every Team In Training event and for all the volunteer duties at the Leukemia & Lymphoma Society and MD Anderson Cancer Center. It was my wall for the Bill Crews Remission Run. Cancer was and is my wall. It is the thing that God put in my heart and mind to do. Build my wall. That's what I am doing.

And whether anyone sees me or I am like the woman picking up trash in the airport, I will build this wall. I have had much opposition. I have been knocked down. I have spent much time in the furnace of affliction. But I have a wall. My wall is cancer. I must build my wall.

"Run when you can, walk if you have to, crawl if you must; just never give up.."

~Dean Karnazes

Chapter 10
The 12th Mile Marker

This tiny book is just a glimpse into my life as an endurance athlete with a wall to destroy and a wall to build. Both of my walls are cancer. I am writing this for my own personal keepsake, but if you happen to come across it, I hope that it helps you to be a bit motivated to keep on moving along in whatever race you're competing in, keeping your eyes on the approaching finish line. It is easy to get so scared that you quit running and take a DNF. If you take a DNF, you don't get the medal around your neck and you miss out on the glory of the finish line. So, if you are out there racing, keep putting one foot in front of the other, slow or fast, until you cross your finish line.

Five young ladies pushed me on at mile 24 in Houston way back in 2006. I hope you can find a way to keep yourself pushing forward when you hit your wall too. You will regret quitting. You will not regret finishing.

I will end with a story about my daughter Morgan who has suffered some of the cruelest of circumstances, yet has chosen over and over to rise from the ashes. At the age of nine, she began asking permission to run a half marathon. I said no and told her to ask again next year. To me, 13 miles is a long distance for a child and she was strong, but very thin. The next year, she asked again and I said no again and told her to ask again when she was 11. So, she did and I said yes. Her first half marathon was in Kingwood, Texas where the finisher medals are the size of Texas. It was so precious seeing her cross the finish line as a tiny 11-year-old and grab that medal that was so heavy it nearly knocked her down. She was hooked.

The next year, at the age of 12, she and I ran the Mardi Gras half marathon in New Orleans together. We wore beads and colorful running skirts and went out with the intention of having fun and dancing at the finish line. At every mile marker along the way, we took a selfie and high-fived each other. After the mile 11 marker, we ran and ran and we struggled greatly. I could see the pain and exhaustion in her face. She kept saying "when will we get to mile 12?" If only I could tell her that I was just as confused. It felt like we were bonking. I pretended to be fine and I tried desperately to keep her calm and focused on running. I wondered if maybe we had gone a bit too fast in the early miles because even I was feeling weighed down. I saw the tears in her sparkling blue eyes and I also saw the fierce determination to keep running. Morgan pushed and pushed and then suddenly, we both looked up and saw mile marker 13! Somehow, we had missed 12 and there we were at 13 with only a sprint to the finish line to go. In an instant, we both started laughing and running fast. The finish line was point one away. And then we saw it. You know the scene, right? I have explained it in previous chapters and all finish lines are the same. Music. Noise of cheering fans. Laughter. Dancing. Food. Medals. Joy. She and I held hands and ran as fast as we could across that finish line and we felt like we had just won gold at the Olympics.

There are moments in life when you miss mile marker 12. I can't explain why that happens. It just does. You might be feeling exhausted and like you cannot take one more step in this heated race. You might even be at a point when you no longer care one ounce about that finish line because all you want to do is quit.

When you miss the mile marker and you have no idea where you are on the course, the temptation to give up becomes profound. You feel like there is nothing left in you to move on and since you don't know how much longer you have, the heat and wind of the race tosses you around in what feels like that furnace of affliction. You hit a wall, a barrier you don't believe you can overcome. Morgan and I were lucky because we had each other when we hit it. As her mom, I had to pretend like everything was fine so that she wouldn't give up, and pretending almost hurts worse than the pain of running and having no idea where you are. The thing I can't forget is how close we were without knowing. If we had quit, we would have regretted it forever. We were right around the corner from the glorious finish line. And, you know what? You might be right around the corner right now from a big victory, so I plead with you, my friend, do not quit!

Today, if you are in agony and no longer want to run, please know that you're not alone. So many others are there too. There are young parents grieving the loss of their child. There are children in hospital beds about to take their last breath. There are people being abused and tormented daily. There are wars. There is poverty and there is hunger. There is great pain out there and billions of people who are suffering. Yes, many want to quit the race as it has gotten unbearable out there. If you need to, take a break and sit on the ground. If you have hit your wall, just stop for a second. Breathe. Cry. Pray. Then, put one foot in front of the other and move forward. If you don't move on, you will miss the glory of the finish line, and who knows how much longer it is? You might have missed mile 12 only to discover that you're much closer than you realized. But no matter what, keep in the race. Cross the finish line and dance.

You might think I am writing this in a moment in my life when I have seen great victory making this so easy to write. But the truth is, I wrote this book on January 3, 2024 with great sorrow. The thing that happened to me at the end of 2023 doesn't really matter. Let's just say that I hit a wall. Actually, it feels more like the giant wall hit me. This one is way too big to climb over and I don't have five adorable young ladies cheering me on. Somehow, I have managed to put a smile on my face when I needed to, but I have cried many tears for days now. I turned 54 last month and I have seen a lot of ugliness in my life. But I have also seen a lot of good. I don't know how far away my finish line is, but I know I won't quit 'til I cross it. I am an endurance athlete. That's what I do.

There is a part of me that is clinging to a tiny bit of hope that I'm about to look up and see mile marker 13 and suddenly feel zeal and joy and be able to run. But I have no idea. Honestly, I have been searching for mile marker 12 for so long now that I want to drop out and never run again.

One of my greatest strengths is determination. Over and over again, I have been forced to make the decision to either quit or push myself and so far, I have always chosen the latter. It might seem strange, but part of the reason I don't want to get Botox is because those wrinkles on my face represent the many times in life when I chose to keep running the race even when I hurt. You see this line on my face? That was my 30-day-old son in a hospital fighting for his life. You see this line? That was my not quite two-year-old daughter falling and fracturing her skull. See this one? That was my husband almost dying of cancer. These are from all the funerals we've attended with those tiny little coffins for precious children who died of cancer. These are from all-night prayer and cry sessions alone in my closet, desperately seeking help. Yes, my wrinkles represent my story and they serve as a reminder to me that life is extremely difficult.

As I search prayerfully and hopefully for mile marker 12, my feet are burning and tears are pouring from my blue eyes and suddenly I realize that for all the glory of the finish line, there is a glory on the race course too. Not knowing how far away I am from that great victory I hope to see, that beautiful finish line which could be miles away or right around the corner, I keep moving. Actually, sometimes I stop for a second to breathe. But then I slowly move forward. That in and of itself is a great glory. The party and all of the celebratory happenings are at the finish line, but there is an incredible glory on the race course too.

You see that guy out there on the Ironman course who is limping along with a mile to go? His limping forward is glory. You see that young mom holding her four-year-old with brain cancer as she takes her final breath? Her love for that child who is about to head into Heaven is glory. You see those men and women and children out there on the course fighting to finish, right? The glory of the finish line is so much more precious when the race course was tough. And trust me, it is tough.

I know that some people have easier race courses. It might seem unfair too because when they cross the finish line, they get a finisher's medal too. And it looks like they didn't have to work as hard or train as hard, so shouldn't we all get medals of different sizes to represent how hard we had to work to get to the finish line? So, the last thought I want to offer is this one. Don't compare. You don't really know what any other runner is experiencing and like Dr. Seuss says "It's a troublesome world. All the people who are in it are troubled with troubles almost every minute."

As a marathon and triathlon coach, I have seen all kinds of stories and struggles. And what I know for sure is that when all the runners line up at the start line, they all kind of look the same. If you take a big step back and just look at them all lined up in their corrals, all you will see are runners. You have no idea what it took to get them to the start line and you have no idea what it will take to get them across the finish line.

I cried some of my happiest and biggest tears seeing my friend Lisa Henthorn cross a finish line in San Antonio because she made her goal time. Most of the people out there that day would not have noticed at all, but her family and friends out there did know. We knew that this was a huge victory for Lisa and we had our very own tear fest and celebration because to us, she might as well have just won a national championship. It took guts for Lisa to even get on the start line and it took a huge depth of strength and determination to get across that finish line in the time she did.

I will never forget one of my Team In Training athletes one morning when she was attempting a 10-mile run in training for her first half marathon. One mile into the training run, she hurt her shins and had to limp back to the park where I was waiting for her. She sat on the ground and starting crying and I don't mean a few little tears. I mean, she was wailing in great agony. Instantly, I wrapped my arms around her and let her tears fall onto my shoulders and then I looked into her eyes and said, "these tears aren't your shins."

No, you see, she had just spent a year fighting her 33-year-old husband's cancer. She had been trying so desperately to be brave and strong for the sake of her children and husband and everyone around her. She did have pain in her shins, just like I had pain in my ankle and knee at the Houston marathon, but shin pain can be overcome much more easily than the grief she was feeling inside. Her wall was blood cancer and it was massive. She just happened to hit it on a training run. I am so glad I experienced being a 33-year-old caregiver to a cancer patient so that I could hold her with compassion and understanding. Ultimately, I got to be part of a great celebration when I saw her cross the finish line in her first half marathon.

And thanks to coaching for Team In Training all those years, I got to see stories like these countless times. I saw young cancer patients fight through their walls and cross finish lines. I saw parents who lost a child to leukemia fight through walls and cross finish lines. I saw folks who had struggled with obesity go out there and fight through walls to cross finish lines (and then lose weight and cross more finish lines). I saw so many victories on race courses that I began to think that everyone should run a marathon just so they could fight their walls and cross finish lines.

Then I realized that everyone is running a marathon. The marathon of life. And in fact, many are doing Ironman and it's dark and the cutoff time is approaching. They have been through cold and dark waters on a swim with waves that nearly drowned them followed by a 112-mile bike through hills and wind and heat. They are out there on their marathon now and they are limping along in great pain. If you see those people, it could be easy to judge them based on the fact that the winner of the race finished hours ago and he's off at the beer tent having fun. You might be thinking that the winner is greater than these losers out here afraid they won't make it by midnight. But let me tell you this. Even the winner is impressed by the last place finisher. I know this from talking to one winner after another.

I used to coach a group of ladies and we called ourselves "Happy Feet" because our feet were happy to be running. On one of our races, we were in San Antonio and they had just run a half marathon and were out walking along the River Walk (or I guess I should say limping). Just ahead of them they spotted the man who won the marathon that day. He was from Africa. He was also limping. He ran the full 26.2-mile marathon faster than they had run the 13.1-mile half marathon. One of the ladies congratulated him and mentioned how embarrassed she was that she was limping when she was so slow and he was so fast and did such a great job. He smiled and told her that they all just run a tough race no matter their pace and they all crossed a finish line that day so they all earned the limping and the medal. I've always loved the fact that true champions are very humble. His pain was likely way more intense than the ladies I was coaching. Running 26 miles at the speed at which he ran causes micro tears in the muscles. He didn't look like he was working hard, but he was working extra hard to make his goal and win the race and trust me, he hurt really bad.

So, when I say "don't compare," I also mean "don't judge." You have no idea what another racer is experiencing. You don't know what it took for them to get to the start line, let alone to the finish line. You don't know about their painful past or current struggles. So, you concentrate on getting yourself to your finish line and encourage those around you on the race course. It's the kind thing to do.

At the Bill Crews Remission Run, we always had a theme for each race. My favorite one was "Celebrate". At packet pickup for that event, a couple in their 50s came in to get their packets and Bill and I were working the table that day. It was perfect because we learned that the husband had been battling the same cancer as Bill and he was not doing well. His precious wife and I had a conversation together while our husbands chatted. An hour later, I was shocked that we were still talking as it seemed like it had only been a few minutes. The next day, the two of them crossed the finish line together in last place. Yes, they were our last finishers. Actually, although they were hand-in-hand, she finished one second ahead of her husband so he was our real last place finisher. So, he not only got a finisher medal, he also got a bottle of champagne to celebrate his finish line victory. And what a victory it was too. He was so weak and frail from chemotherapy that he was lucky not to have to be in a wheelchair that day and there he was walking 3.1 miles to cross a finish line.

Three months later, he took his final breath. His wife joined Team In Training to run a half marathon in his memory and she called me to ask many questions. During our conversation, she began crying and told me that the day her husband and my husband talked at packet pickup was one of the best days she'd had in a long time. She told me that her husband was very closed off about his cancer and never would talk to anyone until he met Bill that day. Apparently, after they left that afternoon, he talked nonstop about his conversation with Bill and how it lifted his spirits. And for the next few months, that champagne at the finish line and his talk with a fellow lymphoma fighter gave him the boost he needed to endure his treatments 'til the end. She was grieved by the loss of her husband and best friend, but she was deeply grateful for the memory of his final three months because he was happy.

The last place finisher deserves a celebration, y'all. At one of my many coaching days with Team In Training, I explained to all the participants that on race day, there will be someone who crosses the finish line first and there will be someone who crosses the finish line last. The rest of us are somewhere in between. I think it helped all of us to remember that we are all on the race course and we are all working at our own abilities and through life circumstances, so no judgment needed. You might be out there wishing you could find mile marker 12 while another person is out there flying past you seemingly pain free. They don't know your struggle and you don't know theirs. You race your race while they race theirs. Get past your wall. Keep moving.

There is a chance that you missed mile marker 12, so please don't quit. I don't know, you could have a long way to go. But no matter what, please don't quit. There is glory on the race course and a celebration at the finish line awaits you. I promise it's there. Don't miss out on that great champagne celebration. Stop and take a few breaths if you need to, but then knock down that big wall and move.

The final theme of our final Bill Crews Remission Run was "The Finish Line." For me, this signified the last time I would host the event, but it also signified the fact that I longed for a finish line in my husband's cancer. You see, his disease continues to be incurable. We have heard a beautiful word for many years and that is what we call in the cancer world "NED" (No Evidence of Disease). But NED is not the same as "cure" and I long to hear that word. Until we hear that word, we remain in the race. In 2014, we discovered another tumor and one of Bill's cancer markers was very high. This came at a time when we were planning to move to Colorado and we had to back out of the job there for a minor surgical procedure to extract the tumor or at least part of it. Bill did not have to begin therapy for this tumor, but he was placed on a watch and wait protocol to monitor its growth and to continue to test the cancer marker. After one year of watching, the tumor shrank and the cancer marker went to a much smaller number. It did not go to normal range until 2019, but thankfully, it was small enough and not spreading so no treatments were necessary.

We will likely never cross a finish line with Bill's cancer. But we won't stop running the race. It is exhausting, but because we learned about the glory of the race course, we stopped being so worried about getting to the finish line. With the advances in treatments, who knows whether we might have just missed mile marker 12 and the finish line is actually only point one away, right? The thing is, we don't know. But we find so much victory and glory in running the race. And surrounding us are people of every age and background. They are running too. They are tired too. We encourage other runners and they encourage us.

I pray for a cure for cancer. I pray for strength to move forward and break down walls every time I hit one. Ultimately, everyone will cross a finish line because you see, we don't live on this planet forever. I know what awaits me at my finish line. My faith is strong enough for me to know that no matter how hard my race is, one day I will cross my ultimate finish line. And just like with Ironman, I will see the big lights at the end of the chute. I will see others who crossed before me cheering as I cross. I will hear the music and see the dancing. I will hear a big booming voice not calling me an Ironman, but saying to me "well done." I will get a crown of glory upon my head. And I will spend eternity celebrating a great victory.

Oh my gosh!!!! I cannot wait. Because I know my finish line is coming, whether I missed that mile marker or not, I will keep putting one foot in front of the other until I cross my finish line. I hope you will too because I can't wait to dance with you there.

"I have fought a good fight.
I have FINISHED the race.
I have kept the faith."

EPILOGUE
The Childhood Cancer Problem

Every day of my life I am immersed in the cancer community and the vast majority of that is the childhood cancer community. What I am about to write here is not a pretty picture, but to honor the kids I fight for, I decided that it needed to be done and this tiny booklet is the right place to do it. You see, when I talk about those walls, it would be wrong not to explain why childhood cancer is a big and seemingly impossible wall.

I realize that the majority of people are not intimately acquainted with pediatric cancer. That's a good thing. I don't want it to be so common that we all understand it. I'm glad that technically, it meets the definition of "rare" and I hope it never becomes common.

But when you are engaged in this tight-knit community of kids with cancer and their families, it feels like childhood cancer is anything but rare. It feels like you are constantly surrounded by sickness and death. It feels like you are screaming your head off trying to get anyone to pay attention to it, but that it is a big act of futility.

I am aware that most people see television ads with adorable little bald kids hanging out with celebrities, or hear about kids getting wish trips to Disney, and the image of childhood cancer becomes "cute". But, please know that childhood cancer is a cruel and hideous monster that is as far from cute as rape or torture of children.

Please know that the analogy I am about to offer might seem evil, but I want you to get this picture in your head because I want you to understand the evil of childhood cancer. If you don't want to read it or think about it, stop now because I'm about to be very bold.

Imagine with me for just a moment a school shooting (I know that is not hard to do since those seem to happen way too frequently). A man with a gun has broken into a school and has shot 50 kids. Seven of those kids are killed while the others are sent to area hospitals to fight for their lives. This not only makes national news. It makes international news doesn't it? Imagine now that it happens again the next day. A shooter walks into a school and shoots 50 kids. Seven die and the others are sent to hospitals to fight for their lives. It happens the next day. And the next. It happens over and over and over again every single day all year long and then the next year, it happens again.

See where I am going? We would be devastated by that kind of loss and we wouldn't say it's "rare". We would be screaming at the top of our lungs for laws and bills and security measures to be in place to end this horror story. Yet, this scene does happen every single day. About 50 children are diagnosed with cancer every day. And seven children die of cancer every day.

By the end of 2024, almost 2,000 kids (people under the age of 20) will die of cancer. Around 16,000 people under the age of 20 will be diagnosed with cancer and begin the fight for their lives that is anything but cute.

Cancer is not just one disease. Cancer is hundreds of diseases and kids suffer much more than adults. The reasons for this are very complex, but the gist of it is that their tiny bodies are still growing and developing and the therapies to try to save their lives are highly toxic. That's right, we are poisoning their tiny growing bodies.

I know many pediatric oncologists and I adore them. What a big calling to have on your life - to try to kill cancer in kids, to see kids dying every day, to fight out there on a battlefield every day where you see massive pain and suffering of babies. Bless everyone who works in pediatric oncology!

When you become a physician, you take an oath to do no harm, so imagine being forced to poison kids. Bless you all.

Several years ago, I met one of my heroes face-to-face and I even was lucky enough to get a big hug from him. His name was Dr. Emil Freireich and he will be forever known as the "father of modern leukemia therapy".

When he came onto the scene back in the beginning of the 1950s, childhood leukemia was 100% fatal. Children were literally bleeding to death on gurneys in hospitals. Blood was pouring out of their eyes and ears and nose and skin. They were lying there in a pool of blood dying and nothing could be done about it.

Dr. Freireich worked with IBM to create a machine that separated the platelets from the blood. He believed that the kids were bleeding to death because of insufficient platelets. This led to the development of the first continuous-flow blood cell separator, for which he holds the patent.

Additionally, he is the one who came up with the idea of treating leukemia in children with combination chemotherapy, in which cancer drugs are given simultaneously rather than singly. He also believed in a holistic approach to treating these children. Today, the five-year survival rate for children with acute lymphocytic leukemia, the most common childhood leukemia, is about 90% overall. If you would like to know more about this incredible hero of mine, I recommend heading to the MD Anderson website to read more or even better, pick up a copy of the book *Cancer, The Emperor of All Maladies* by Siddhartha Mukheriee. The book became a documentary film done in three parts and it can be viewed now on PBS.

I actually met Dr. Freireich at a screening of the film. He was wheelchair-bound by then, but still working hard as a physician at MD Anderson. Some people get excited to meet movie stars and rock stars. I was excited to meet this doctor as if he were the biggest celebrity on the planet. Men like these are true heroes. I reached my hand out to shake his hand when my friend Erika said "he's a germaphobe" (which of course made me love him more since I am too). Instead of a handshake, I got a hug. I had a short, yet lovely chat with the man who spent his life saving children's lives and I will never forget that honor. He died in 2020, but his legacy lives on and every child who has fought leukemia can thank him for his breakthroughs that led to their life-saving therapies.

Now, having said all that, no one wants to have to give chemotherapy agents to any person of any age, but especially kids. Sure, chemo can kill cancer cells, but it also kills healthy cells. Among the kids who survive leukemia, almost all of them are left with vast side effects and late effects including infertility, rotting out teeth, damage to their heart and other internal organs, increased risk for developing secondary and third cancers and much more.

Research is crucial. Not only do we need to learn more about how malignancies develop in kids, but we also need to work hard to develop better therapies, therapies that kill cancer cells while leaving normal, healthy cells alone. And, this is being done. It is costly and it is very time-consuming.

In addition to the nightmare of leukemia, there are still today cancers in kids that are almost 100% fatal. Diffuse intrinsic pontine glioma (DIPG) is a brain cancer in kids. There are a handful of teenage patients who have survived past the two-year mark, but most of the patients are under the age of 11 and they die within a year. And these deaths are extremely cruel. These kids soon become "trapped in their bodies". They can hear everything happening around them and they can see. They are fully aware of their surroundings, but they cannot talk or move and then eventually, they can no longer breathe. It is a merciless disease.

Every year, Bill and I attend CureFest for Childhood Cancer in Washington, D.C. CureFest is held during National Childhood Cancer Awareness Month (September). Its mission is to make childhood cancer research a national priority by uniting the childhood cancer community, the general public and government officials as one voice against childhood cancer. Following the COVID pandemic, CureFest increased its reach with an in-person event in Washington, D.C. and a virtual event held in 68 countries. It is live-streamed for anyone who cannot attend.

Bill and I attend as part of the National Advisory Council with Gold Together for Childhood Cancer at American Cancer Society. Ahead of the weekend events, Gold Together sends ambassadors, both young and old, to speak to legislators about important bills we need passed as well as increased funding for pediatric cancer. Advocacy is extremely important.

When President Richard Nixon first signed the National Cancer Act in 1971, officially declaring war on cancer, our federal government began funding cancer research. Sadly, of all the funding, less than 4% of that was allocated to childhood cancer research and this persisted for decades. Finally, in 2021, a great breakthrough happened. Congress heard our cries and now more than 8% of federal funds are allocated to childhood cancer. This is thanks in large part to the Congressional Childhood Cancer Caucus, a bipartisan caucus co-chaired by Representative Michael McCaul and Representative Chris Van Hollen. Their mission is to work together to address pediatric cancer, advocate in support of measures to prevent the pain, suffering and long-term effects of childhood cancers, and to work toward the goal of eliminating cancer as a threat to all children.

I am grateful to be one of the voices for these kids. When we speak with our representatives, both at the state and federal levels, we know they listen. How could they not? Sure, they fight about every other topic under the sun, but when it comes to childhood cancer, it doesn't matter how far they are on the left or on the right, they meet in unity when it comes to these kids.

In addition to federal funds, I know from years of hard work, that the problem of childhood cancer cannot be solved with the government alone. Philanthropy is the answer and we must have more people willing to open their hearts and wallets to end these diseases. I am so honored to serve as a volunteer with Gold Together. We are currently funding 49 different multi-year research grants in the amount of $29 million. I don't know if I will get to see the end of cancer as a threat to kids in my lifetime, but when I take my final breath, I hope that I will realize that the work I committed myself to in this life was at least a small part of bringing these diseases to an end.

I know this book was not about childhood cancer. But also, it was. You see, as I mentioned, it is my wall. It is my wall to destroy - to see the complete eradication of childhood cancer. It is also my wall to build - to see a protective wall around these kids, a wall to shut out the evil and enclose them in something powerfully good.

My friends, if you made it this far into the epilogue, I urge you to get involved in the fight against childhood cancer. I remember for the longest time seeing a sea of pink in October, whether I was at a football game or the shopping mall. Pink was everywhere. One year, my son came home from school when he was in the 5th grade with an armband that read "I love boobies". Honestly, that was inappropriate to me, but that's not the point. The point is that his school had hosted a "paint the path pink" event for breast cancer. I am not mad that breast cancer gets attention. Way too many people get breast cancer and I lost two close friends to it when they were in their 40s. I absolutely want an end to breast cancer!

I see the effects of turning everything pink in October. It led to better awareness and funding to cure breast cancer. I don't want to stop seeing pink. What I want to see changed is that I also get to see more gold. I don't want this to happen due to more kids getting diagnosed. Instead, I want to see way more allies in this war on childhood cancer. I want to see people who have never known a child with cancer put on their gold, head out to speak to legislators, donate to research, and get involved in the fight to end childhood cancer.

So, I ask you to join me as I destroy the wall that blocks us from the cures and I ask you to help me build a wall of protection. As you fight your good fight and work to finish your race, will you please consider racing with me and the precious little kids who need us?

Today, there will be small children taking their final breath. Their race in life was too short and it was violently painful. I plead with you, my friend, put on your gold and fight because children are more precious than gold and they need us.

My email address is dcrews@bellasteri.com and I am here to answer the questions you might have and help guide you to many ways you can help these kids and their families. I look forward to hearing from you and I thank you in advance for having a heart of gold.

Thank you for reading this little booklet. Thank you for running your race at whatever pace you're running it. Thank you for choosing to move forward no matter how hard you might have hit your wall. Whatever your calling is, go fulfill it. Be blessed. As you get closer and closer to the finish line, you will have good moments and you will have painful moments. Keep your faith. I will see you at the finish line.

Love and blessings,
DS

About the Author

Dana-Susan Crews lives in Fort Worth, Texas with her husband Bill and her miniature schnauzer Bella. She is an author and public speaker who continues to love swimming and running (but not cycling).

She has worked for and volunteered for many nonprofit organizations including MD Anderson Cancer Center, the Leukemia & Lymphoma Society, Lymphoma Research Foundation, and American Cancer Society. She is the owner and co-founder of Bell Asteri Publishing & Enterprises, LLC and an advocate for childhood cancer. She serves on the National Advisory Council for Gold Together for Childhood Cancer and is an active member of the Coalition Against Childhood Cancer.

She can be contacted at dcrews@bellasteri.com

Other Books by the Author

A Time to Fight (second edition)
Our Daddy's Cancer
Chemo Dates
Surviving Someone Else's Cancer, A Journal for Caregivers
Cancer Warrior Journal (for siblings of kids with cancer)
My Mommy Has Cancer (explaining cancer to kids)
My Daddy Has Cancer (explaining cancer to kids)

Find all of the above at your favorite bookstore or visit www.bellasteri.com

www.ingramcontent.com/pod-product-compliance
Lightning Source LLC
LaVergne TN
LVHW052341080426
835508LV00045B/3219